What parents and experts are saying about

Nurturing Baby and Me During Pregnancy

" An elegant book with valuable measures to pleasurably strengthen the parental bond"
—**Dr. Clark Gillespie, M.D.,** American College of Obstetricians and
Gynecologists Life Fellow and author of *Your Pregnancy Month by Month.*

"Nurturing Baby and Me During Pregnancy is a vital concept presented in a refreshing, rewarding method."
—**Dr. Richard Crandall III,** Family Physician, *Landisville, PA.*

"…especially good for women who may have ambivalent feelings or little support. The parent's stories share good insights and the journal helps get out true feelings."
—**Angela Bonner, RN,** Childbirth and Breastfeeding Educator, *Irving, Texas*

" This program will help make parents more confident and give them coping and relaxing skills for after baby arrives."
—**Jennifer Wilson, BA, LBSW,** Parenting and Child Development Teacher,
Spirit Lake, Iowa.

" …the exercises helped me shift my focus from the pain to imagining my baby and it always puts a smile on my face."
—**Elena D,** *New Britain, CT*

Nurturing Baby and Me During Pregnancy

by Arlene Matthews, MA
Susan Fekety, MSN, CNM

Designed by Debra Tremper
and Lisa Collins

Developing Hearts Systems, Inc.
Stratford, Connecticut

ISBN-13: 978-1-59975-135-1
ISBN-10: 1-59975-135-6

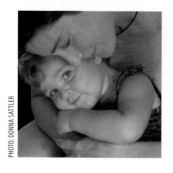

How using this program will
make you an even better parent

THE TOOLS AND TECHNIQUES in this book will show you how to start reaching out to your baby during pregnancy and get ready for a life together. You'll learn…

» **Scientists are starting to gather information about things that women have suspected for a long time.** For centuries, women of many cultures have interacted with their unborn children. Although we'll never know what unborn babies "think" or "feel," it does appear that they notice more about their world than we used to think. Stay tuned!

» **Parenting starts while you're pregnant.** What you do now with your body and the one growing inside you prepares you for your role as a parent. Find out how pregnancy is the best time to prepare yourself, before the challenges of infant care.

» **The most important factor in parenting is love and the time to love.** Learn how to take quiet time, relax, and use music and tested techniques to send love to your unborn child.

By using this book you will develop the ability:

» **To be more confident and ready.** You'll hear stories from women who overcame their fears and found strength by focusing on getting to know their babies before birth.

» **To benefit you and your baby by practicing the art of relaxation.** You'll learn how a few minutes a day can actually reduce your stress hormones and help you have a healthier pregnancy. And it feels good!

» **To start reaching out now.** When baby is born – you'll feel like you've always known your child!

Who can use this program

First-time parents	This book provides a gentle and engaging introduction to the possibilities, responsibilities, and joys of having a child.
Already parents	Helps experienced parents have a more easy-going and rewarding pregnancy and a close relationship with their child.
Fathers and family	This book shows a dad-to-be and others how to get involved from day one.
Single moms-to-be	It will help you build the inner strength and confidence needed to raise a healthy and happy child.
Gift givers	Give a gift of love to your mom-to-be and her baby. Know too that part of your purchase goes to helping moms in need through our non-profit service partners.
Family Service/ Healthcare Providers	This tool can help make your programs and services more effective by supporting healthy family development at the earliest possible opportunity. Please see bondingwithbaby.org for how our non-profit publishing agency provides our books at the lowest possible cost to qualified providers.

Contents

Foreword

Having a baby these days can have its stressful moments. Health researchers continue to see the adverse affects of that stress on a pregnant woman's body, her baby, and her important relationships.

Supporting a woman to relax, enjoy pregnancy as a natural process and prepare mentally for parenthood is as important as good prenatal care. This is where the experienced and gentle hand of a certified nurse-midwife or certified midwife can ease both the physical and emotional journey of pregnancy.

Unfortunately, your midwife can't be with you 24 hours a day, but the physical and psychological benefits that come with a regular practice of emotional relaxation are the next best thing! Special tools, like the Nurturing Baby and Me During Pregnancy program, provide easy and enjoyable exercises you can use to release your daily stressors.

This program will engage your inner spirit and help you begin to connect with your baby and grow in ways you didn't think you could. Midwives know that these early bonds set the stage for the emotional health of your family. So take an active role! Join us and start enjoying your pregnancy as you prepare to enjoy your new baby.

—**Deanne Williams,** CNM Executive Director, American College of Nurse-Midwives

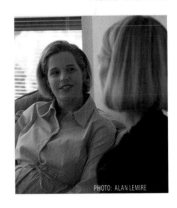

PHOTO: ALAN LEMIRE

Acknowledgments

The publisher gives thanks to the **Freddie Mac Foundation** for funding the development and distribution of this book. We also extend our gratitude to **Healthy Families America,** who collaborated with us to bring it to their families in need. A big thanks also goes to the **American College Of Nurse-Midwives** who offered the book to their members and moms-to-be. A special thanks to all the ground-breakers in prenatal parenting, including **Drs. Rene Van de Carr, David Chamberlain and Thomas Verny,** who founded the **Association for Pre- and Perinatal Psychology and Health** and whose pioneering work enabled us to create this practical guidebook to help new families.

A big thank you goes to **Drs. Glade Curtis, Clark Gillespie** and **Richard Crandall III,** and to **Angela Bonner, RN, Jennifer Wilson, LBSW,** and Certified Nurse-Midwives **Katy Despot, Eliza Holland** and **Amanda Skinner** for their review and kind words. And a special thanks to **Dr. William and Martha Sears** for their encouragement and contribution.

Thanks to the **General Electric Medical Systems** for the generous donations of sonogram images. We'd also like to thank all the parents who contributed their photos, stories and ideas for this book and invite all readers to send in their experiences for the next one.

Thanks to **Sharon Castlen** of **Integrated Book Marketing** for guiding us through the book-publishing maze.

A personal note: This program is dedicated to my Mom, **Jenny Sullivan,** who died before she saw what she inspired.

Tom Berquist,
Executive Director
Developing Hearts Systems
A non-profit educational publisher

Contributors

Proofreading by Jeanmarie Martin, awaywithwords.name and Tina Puckett.

Researchers: Brooke Huntley, Erika Jones, and Peggy Schwende.

Research Assistance: Becky Hagadorn Catamount Group, BabytoBe.com and Firm Facts.

Writers/Interviewers: Charlie Arnett, Rachel Davis, Genesa Garbarino, Rebecca Holladay, Audra Nelson, Donna Nichols, September Sannes, Susan Zemelman.

Writers: Kimberly Metera, Mary Zhou

Photographers: Carmen Ciobanu, Andrew Collings andrewcollings.com, Cara Garbarino, Alan Lemire alanlemire.com, Donna Sattler, amothersimage.com, Jon Okuma, and Roger Salls, rogersallsphtography,com

Graphic Design: Debra Tremper sixpennygraphics.com, and Lisa Collins

The many parents who shared their time, pictures and stories: Megan and Eoin Clarke, Andrina Dacosta, Kathleen Cassidy and Aaron Sojourner, Alli Zaro Fitzgerald, Dominique Ndome Minoue, Alicia Murchison, Maggie & Stella Formato, Lavonna Tunstall, Kristy Zukeran, Maggie and Stella Formato.

Recording: Robert Potterton III, composer and recording artist, Fred Rosamundo and Lee Walkup at Grace Recording Studios, Helen Little of *Little Voices,* Jamil Holyfield at Radio One Philadelphia and Grekim Jennings.

Healthy Families America collaborators: Barbara Rawn, Helen Reif, Johanna Schuchert, Teresa Morewitz and numerous staff and family support workers who made this possible.

The many people who have helped our non-profit over the years: Bill Colrus, Ray Leibman, Kent Wahlberg, Ken Fassman, Seme Ndzana, Marie Roker, Crystal Astrachan, Maurice Segall and the ProBono Partnership.

Introduction:
Benefits of an early start

Advances in prenatal technology and brain science research are changing how we think about pregnancy and the womb world. We are only beginning to explore whether, and if so how, babies can sense, feel and learn during the prenatal period. Early evidence suggests that the unborn are more aware than many of us thought.

This book is designed to help you know some special ways to love and get to know your new family member, and how to have a more peaceful and relaxed pregnancy. Our program will introduce you to stress-reduction techniques, visualization and breathing exercises, stimulation of the fetus through music, talking and touch, and ways to involve the baby's father in the pregnancy journey.

Though it's tough to draw firm scientific conclusions in this area yet, it's interesting to think about whether a program in prenatal enrichment can help babies to get the best start in life. What's important is to start your journey knowing you are parents already.

In places where programs like this one have been tried (see the Resource List at the back of the book for more information), researchers felt they saw benefits such as these:

Benefits For Mothers
» Were better able to handle labor
» Had greater success at breastfeeding
» Felt more attuned to baby's signals and needs
» Were more confident as a parent

Benefits For Baby
» Enhanced motor development
» Enhanced language development
» Earlier social engagement (smiling, playing peek-a-boo)
» More content and better able to control emotions

Benefits For Family
» Showed greater bonding
» Provided greater family cohesion

Benefits of Love
This book is not about creating "super babies." It's not even about the wonders of science or nature at work. This book is about the magic of a mother's (and father's) love at work. It is your dedication to the practice of becoming a good parent which will allow this book to yield practical benefits for you and your child.

Parenting starts during pregnancy

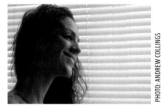

You've probably already heard stories from parents (like those in our book) who've talked with their babies in the womb. Perhaps you're a bit skeptical about whether you can do this too, or if you'll notice the same sorts of things.

All babies are different – but the love bond is universal. Enjoy it!

Preparing for a new child is no longer just about eating right, getting enough rest, and preparing the nursery. If you're already pregnant, your baby is in constant communication with you, receiving signals about the world through your body and the love you send every day.

Mothers know that parenting starts during pregnancy. Everything you need to learn to become a good parent, you can start learning and doing before your baby is born:

» Providing a safe, secure, and relaxed home environment in the womb

» Becoming a tuned-in caregiver able to appreciate and respond to baby's moods and activities

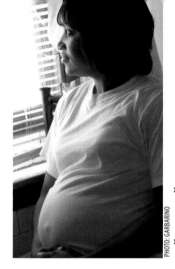

PHOTO: GARBARINO

» Stimulating healthy growth through interactions that may support baby's development

» Beginning the important bonding process so baby grows up trusting and confident

Pregnancy is an ideal time to pause and take the opportunity to practice parenting. Before you know it, baby will be there in your arms.

Learning to parent your unborn child is simple—and the joys and benefits are enormous. Start by believing you can. Take a few minutes each day to learn how and practice nurturing yourself and your unborn. Try it. Tap your tummy and say, *"I'm right here, baby."*

Program Basics

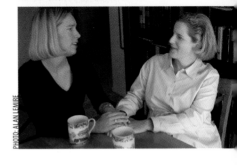

PHOTO: ALAN LEMIRE

This program helps you and your baby in three basic ways:

Physical

We live in stressful times. Pregnancy can add considerably more stress, and stress can cause complications in pregnancy.

Starting with the first month and continuing throughout pregnancy, our Quiet Time exercises and special music will help you lower your stress levels. Overall, pregnancy, labor, and the birth process all seem to go better when a mom is relaxed. Maybe someday science will show what many moms suspect – that when they're relaxed, they send "feel good" messenger molecules to their babies to say the world is safe and love will be abundant.

Psychological

By doing the various exercises, you will learn to become more confident during pregnancy and a more in-tune parent.

You'll be doing journal-writing exercises that will encourage you to express and accept your feelings, which make you more ready to handle the challenges ahead.

You'll learn the technique of replacing negative thoughts with positive affirmations, and gain a greater sense of control over your changing life. By frequently affirming your faith and hopes, you become an empowered parent more ready and able to do this important job.

Interactive

You've been interacting with your baby on a physical level since conception. As baby gets older and its senses develop more fully, you'll come to experience that your baby can hear, feel and sometimes even respond to you. This book and CD will help you take advantage of this two-way communication by learning to stimulate and nurture your baby through words, sound, songs, movement, and touch.

Easy Program Steps

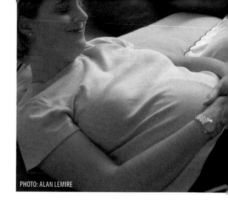

Each week you can…

1. Look forward to what's in store for you and your baby for the week.

2. Learn something new about your developing baby.

3. See a sonogram of babies at your child's stage and visualize what your baby may look like.

4. Understand your continuing role in nurturing your unborn child and helping your baby grow.

5. Learn what other new families have done to bond with their unborn children.

6. Take a daily Quiet Time breather and listen to soothing music to release stress.

7. Do a coach-guided exercise that will help you gain self-awareness and feel closer to your new baby each day.

Tips for the Best Start

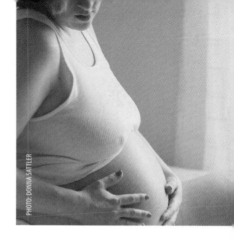

Let your Pregnancy Coach guide you.

The exercises and music on the CD were specifically developed to relax and gently guide you. Wherever you find this CD symbol, play that track. It will make your experience more fulfilling and more fun.

» **Promise yourself** you will reserve at least 15 minutes each day for you and baby to take a Quiet Time break and do the daily exercise.

» **Start at the beginning.** No matter when you receive this book, review the objectives in the first chapters and get used to the beginning exercises before you go forward. This will help you ease into the program. If you don't feel ready for an exercise, maybe try it again later. Don't stress yourself about trying to catch up!

» **Don't rush ahead.** This program works one step at a time and builds in stages. Stay in the moment with your baby and don't be impatient. The rest of your pregnancy will unfold quickly enough. It's okay to work backwards in the book, but don't skip ahead.

» **Be natural.** As soon as you feel you want to start sending loving thoughts to your baby –go ahead! It's always the right time to love your baby.

PHOTO: DONNA SATTLER

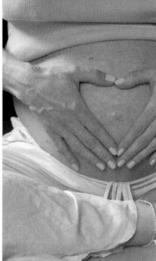

focus

» **Go with your feelings.** If you and baby enjoy certain exercises more than others –do more of them. If you don't enjoy some or feel they aren't good for baby, skip them. YOU are in charge.

» **Stay with it.** Sometimes you'll be repeating an exercise over a period of weeks. For you and baby to derive the full benefit, it's best to keep practicing.

» **Take your Quiet Time any-where/anytime you can focus on baby.** You don't have to be lying down in your bedroom to do many of the exercises. Some might work for you in your parked car at lunch or while riding a bus. Quiet Time works anytime your mind can focus to devote your attention and feelings toward your baby.

» **Take it gentle and easy.** Do not over-stimulate your baby or try and crowd more exercises into a shorter period. More is not better and will not create a "baby genius." Your baby spends most of his time sleep-ing – that's Mother Nature's plan!

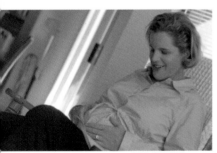

PHOTO: ALAN LEMIRE

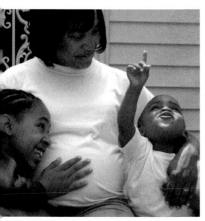

PHOTO: GARBARINO

» **Consult your healthcare provider.** Although there is nothing unsafe about doing the exercises in this program, let your doctor or midwife know what you are doing just in case there's an unusual circumstance or concern.

» **Relax.** You are a busy woman these days with a lot on your mind. Don't worry about skipping an exercise here and there or staying on a strict schedule. Relax and have fun.

» **Respect your traditions.** You may not be comfortable with all the exercises in this book. If they do not fit with your cultural, religious or family traditions, don't do them—or adapt them to your own beliefs. If you are a person with strong religious beliefs, as you do these exercises feel free to imagine the warm glow of love as your God or any other higher power that you believe in.

» **Remember that babies develop at different rates and have different temperaments.** If baby doesn't respond to a certain activity how and when it says in the book, don't worry. Everyone's different, and that includes babies! Some may not kick back or seem to want to play. There's no "right way" for a baby to behave. Try the exercise later, or just skip it. Still – trust your intuition: if you ever feel there is something wrong with your baby, check in with your midwife or doctor as soon as you can.

A word about fathers, family and single parenting

Think of ways you can get your partner involved in baby's development. Read these introductory pages together. Show him the pictures and stories of other dads who enjoyed participating. Listen to the CD together – relaxing is good for both of you! Tell him he'll be able to hear his baby's heartbeat when he joins you at a prenatal visit. Play the kick game as a family. Tell him that if he talks to his baby every day, the day baby is born the baby will recognize his voice.

You need all the help you can get. Even though you will be doing most of the "heavy lifting," having helpful people involved with you in this program will make your pregnancy more enjoyable.

Fathers. There are lots of ways a dad-to-be can help and your new family will benefit. By getting Dad involved in doing many of the exercises with you, he'll get used to the idea that you'll be spending lots of time with baby. You'll not only lessen any resentment that he may be feeling, but you'll inspire him to become much more involved in the care-giving. By gaining a better understanding of your pregnancy and learning with you, he will become more sensitive to your needs and help you keep your stress level

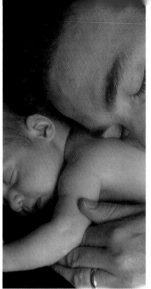

PHOTO: DONNA SATTLER

down. An early-engaged father or partner will start building the bonds of your family.

A strong relationship between fathers and babies helps children do better on developmental assessments, be happier and better able to handle frustrations, and overall have better self-esteem while they grow up. Together as a family, you will make parenthood more meaningful.

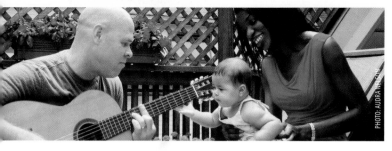

Get others involved now for you and baby.

Those important others. The more social and emotional support you are lucky enough to find, the better. If you have other children, you'll see they can participate in the program too –and it will make them more ready to be a good big brother or sister. Beyond important family members, you can ask a trusted friend or non-judgmental minister or counselor to listen to your problems and give you emotional support. Doulas, nurses, and midwives can also be excellent sources of support and prenatal preparation.

Single parenting

Having said all that about father involvement, that may not be possible for you. Not every pregnant woman reading this book will be in a committed relationship. Like every new parent, you will want to look at the situation into which your baby will be born and create the best supportive environment you can. Do not feel that your child will be a deprived child. You don't have to be burdened with guilt and you don't have to go it alone. Talk to your health care provider for help.

Look for social services or family support agencies in your area. Try to find a support group or prenatal class in the phone book or in your community center, church or library. This book will help give you the confidence and tools to help get you started parenting. Remember: Millions of single women are out there single parenting and doing an excellent job. You can too.

Your partner. Although your helper could be a friend or family member, male or female, we're going to refer to whomever you find to help you with the exercises as your partner or the baby's dad. Feel free to translate!

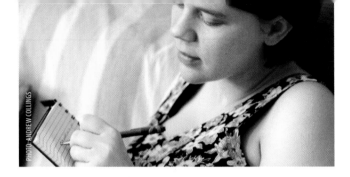

PHOTO: ANDREW COLLINGS

A word about journal writing…

This is one of the most helpful exercises you'll be doing throughout the program. Don't worry if you're not familiar with it or feel you're not much of a writer. Journal writing is simply about getting your inner thoughts and feelings out and on paper. Think of it as a diary—which no one else has to ever see—where writing down important thoughts gives you a sense of relief and makes things clearer to you.

A word about affirmations…

For the reader who may not be familiar with this powerful technique, think of the children's picture book, The Little Engine That Could. By saying "I think I can" over and over again with each stroke of his engine, the little locomotive was able to find the courage and power to climb mountains. Affirmations help you get a picture in your mind of you already doing and being the best that you can do and be. They're like a road map from the idea to the real thing. Affirmations give you inner power to meet the challenges you face.

For each period of your pregnancy, we're going to give you some suggestions on the kind of affirmations that could be helpful, but you'll also want to create your own. Discover what matters most to you, find inspiring words, and speak them from the heart. Affirmations—with your feelings and faith behind them—will empower you to become the best mother you can be.

All that journal writing requires is that you be open and honest with yourself and let yourself flow with whatever words come to mind—even just a word or two. We'll be guiding you with little prompts that get you started. Journal-writing can help you uncover issues that need addressing and create messages of hope and love for your baby.

Let's get clear about pregnancy milestones—months and weeks!

It's easy to get confused about all the different ways "pregnancy time" is measured. Pregnancy lasts 10 lunar months, but these are not the same as months on a calendar. Your doctor or midwife measures your pregnancy in weeks from your last menstrual period, but that includes a couple weeks when you weren't even pregnant yet. Scientists who study how babies grow talk about how old they are from the time of conception, which won't match up with the number of weeks from your period. And then your friend wants to know how many "months along" you are, and you count it out and divide by four – and it doesn't work right. Yikes! It's a pretty crazy system!

To keep things simple, this program uses a calendar based on how many weeks have passed since your last menstrual period, since that's what your prenatal care is based on. We'll also tell you the trimester you're in, and how many lunar months have passed since your period. But we advise you to stick with counting in weeks. Your doctor or midwife will always be able to tell you how many weeks along you are. Your baby's developmental age will be a couple of weeks less than that.

Here's the important message: don't worry about exact dates. (We know you have better things to do!) Just notice the approximate times your baby is developing in different ways. She's on her own schedule, and that's just as it should be!

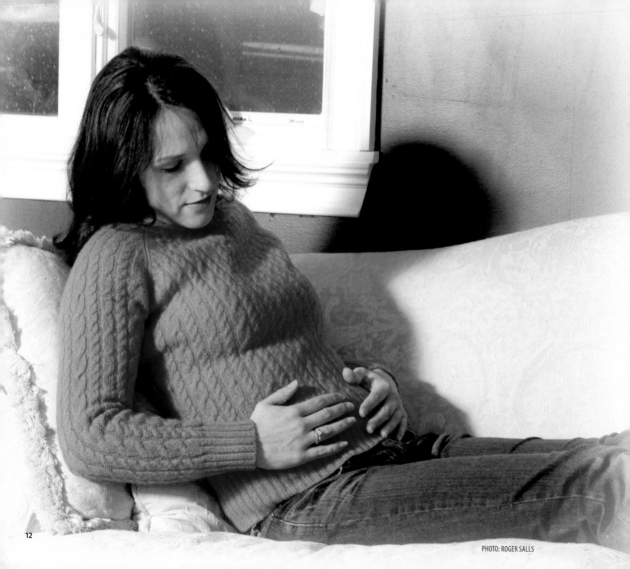

12

Month 1 Goal:
Learn and enjoy doing a Quiet Time exercise every day.

Week 1 Objective:
Record your feelings about being pregnant.

My Pregnancy Journal

For part (maybe all!) of this month you didn't know you were pregnant. But then – the big news came. If you are like most women, you had some mixed feelings when you learned you were pregnant. It's really normal for a part of you to feel you're not ready for this! Write out your first feelings and thoughts about how you felt when you found out you were pregnant. (Use the blank pages in the back of this book, or a separate journal.)

When I first found out, I wondered: _____

_____

I was most excited about:

_____

_____

Now that I am pregnant, I will take better care of myself by:

_____

_____

A Parent's Experience

"I tried to take care of myself better, tried to get a lot of sleep, tried to let a lot of stresses not bother me. For the first time in my life, I tried to care for myself emotionally and physi-cally. For the first time, what other people wanted didn't matter so much anymore. Even though I was young, I no longer cared about peer pressure, I just did what was best for the baby at that point."

Vicki T. and Kevin
– Illinois

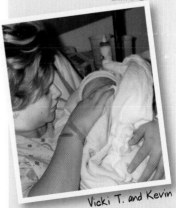

Vicki T. and Kevin

Week 2 Objective:

Understand the importance of managing stress.

Providing a good womb environment and reducing stress

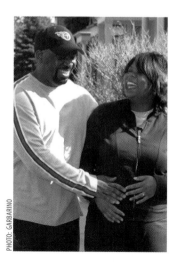

Stress is your body's reaction to a situation that requires a response from you, either physical (like running away, or slamming on the brakes in your car) or emotional (like being nervous, or embarrassed, or sad.) In times of stress, our body releases several hormones and chemicals that help us to respond by increasing our heart rate, blood pressure, muscle tension and breathing. Ordinarily, our bodies are good at bringing themselves back to a relaxed state after our reaction, but when we experience long periods of stress, these hormones can be found at high levels in our blood.

There is lots of research accumulating in the medical world which shows that stress hormones can trigger body changes in you that affect your pregnancy health. (See the Resources List.) A certain amount of stress during pregnancy is normal, of course, but learning some positive ways of managing uncomfortable amounts of stress can benefit both you and your baby.

There are many good relaxation techniques such as yoga and breathing exercises that can really help you handle your stress better. Many pregnant women have found that breathing exercises help them to feel calmer and more relaxed. You will probably learn some of these techniques later on in your pregnancy when you take childbirth classes, but you can go ahead and practice relaxing right now!

Week 3 Objective:

Learn, practice, and enjoy taking a daily Quiet Time break.

Find your stress-reducer.

This program features a specially developed series of Quiet Time activities to reduce stress in moms-to-be. In addition, exercise, hobbies, and simply unwinding– shopping with a girlfriend or watching TV – can provide good relaxation. Take the time now to develop a regular stress-reduction routine for your pregnancy.

What's Quiet Time?

Quiet Time is a simple guided breathing and visualization routine that puts your mind and body into a relaxed, peaceful state. This routine, practiced regularly, could become a valuable stress-reducer for you and a well-deserved break from the pressures of the day. Taking a daily "Quiet Time" puts you in closer touch with your feelings and with your baby, reduces stress, and makes you feel refreshed and more confident afterwards. On the next page, there are ten steps to gently guide you along a beautiful path to physical and emotional relaxation (sometimes with the help of a partner), bringing you to a quiet, wonderful place. Daily Quiet Time is a cornerstone of our program and its effectiveness. This routine will carry through after the baby's birth and we predict that it will continue to be your favorite time together.

How do I get started?

» Look at your daily schedule and find the best slot for taking 15 minutes every day.

» Let your family know you need to take this Quiet Time for yourself and not be disturbed for 15 minutes. Make sure any other children are attended and tell your family they will participate later.

» Find a quiet, private spot where you can get comfortable, such as a bedroom. Take the phone off the hook and lock the door if you have to.

» Lie on your side on a bed or find a chair that you're comfortable in, get ready to relax, and turn to step 1>

Learn the Quiet Time steps by heart, practice every day, and experience letting go of stress.

10 steps to a successful Quiet Time

1. From a comfortable position, let your body relax, and take three or four slow, deep breaths. Let each breath fill up your abdomen and move up into your chest.

 Track 1

2. Close your eyes and take three or four more deep breaths; focus on breathing out until you feel a natural rhythm.

3. As you breathe and feel your body relaxing, start paying attention to your body and mind.

4. Start thinking of your toes, then your feet, and start to move slowly up your body one part at a time—pausing for a moment to see if it feels tight or full of tension.

5. Each time you encounter a part that feels tense, use your outgoing breath to release the tension. Feel it flowing out as your body part becomes limp and relaxed.

6. Keep slowly moving up your body from legs to torso to arms and shoulders and release any tension you find with your outgoing breaths.

7. When you reach your head, begin to relax your face starting with your eyebrows, then your eyes, down to your mouth and feel your whole jaw relax. Then release all of the tensions and worries you find in your mind and let your head and your whole body sink into a soft, warm position.

8. In your mind, slowly repeat: "Calm and peaceful, peaceful and warm" for one minute.

9. Picture yourself in a favorite place from your past or from your imagination—a place where it is safe and warm. Stay in that place with that feeling for a minute.

10. In your mind, repeat to yourself several times, "I am relaxed and I am ready." Then open your eyes and slowly return to your daily activities.

Week 4 Objective:

Continue your daily Quiet Time and create an affirmation that motivates you to take time each day until baby is born.

Your decision and action is required.
We know how tough it is today for a busy woman, let alone a pregnant one, to find time to relax. But if you want to give yourself and your baby the best benefits of this program, you will want to commit to it and do it every day. Use your Quiet Time breaks this week to see yourself releasing all doubts and excuses you might have about not taking the time.

Create an affirmation—a promise to yourself how you're going to be or do the best you can—to take this time for yourself and baby. Some examples:

"I am taking Quiet Time to get closer every day to my baby." "I am helping my baby and me grow stronger during Quiet Time."

My Pregnancy Journal

Today, I promised myself and my baby that I will take a Quiet Time break every day.

Signed: _____

I chose these words as my affirmation: _____

_____

_____

Say your affirmation out loud each day before you take your Quiet Time and say it out loud in front of the mirror every night before you go to bed and each morning when you get up.

FIND time to *relax*

PHOTO: DONNA SATTLER

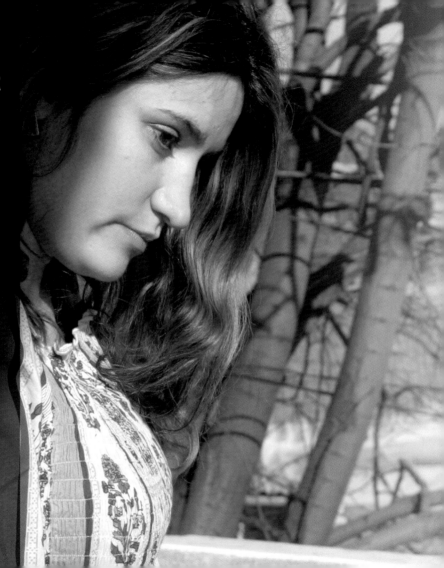

THE NEED TO ADDRESS YOUR FEELINGS.

Having a new baby requires many changes in your life that can cause you to worry or even doubt yourself. If negative feelings persist they can take away the enjoyment of this special time and the stress could affect your health. Take this week to understand the importance of stress reduction.

Month 2 Goal:
Explore and express feelings that could lead to stress.

Week 5 Objective:
Understand how stress can affect your baby.

Potential effect of chronic stress on your baby

The placenta you will be growing for your new baby provides everything needed for proper growth. It acts like a lung to provide oxygen and a digestive system for the intake of food and removal of waste. As a mother, you can provide the best environment for your baby by having a healthy lifestyle, eating the right foods, and getting plenty of rest.

Your baby's growth is not only affected by food and exercise, but also by what you think and feel, because feelings can cause reactions in your body. Pregnancy is a time full of changes and emotions.

When pregnant women are under lots of stress for long periods, it is thought that this can interfere with the amount of nutrients available to their unborn children, and potentially result in babies who are small at birth or born prematurely.

There's little point in getting stressed about being stressed! Just be aware that you can do a lot to lessen the negative impact of stress for you.

Week 6 Objective:

Express your feelings about being pregnant.

My Pregnancy Journal

How have things changed since pregnancy?

_____

_____

How does my family feel about my pregnancy?

_____

_____

My two biggest hopes for the future:

1. _____

2. _____

My two TOP concerns about my pregnancy:

1. _____

2. _____

Two things I'm feeling confident about:

1. _____

2. _____

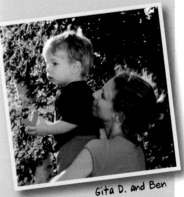

Gita D. and Ben

Week 7 Objective:

Use Quiet Time to uncover any negative feelings.

By now you've become accustomed to using your Quiet Time to reduce stress and relax. Now you'll use this technique to identify your feelings about being pregnant. As you know, inner feelings can find their way into the body, like with a muscle tension or a blush, so you're going to now listen to your body and to what it tells you.

NOTE: These exercises involve exploring your inner feelings. If you are not comfortable doing that, skip them. Or, if you find yourself feeling uncomfortable, stop or consider seeking the help of a counselor.

This week you'll start your Quiet Time as before. Follow steps 1-4 on page 16 and pause at any body part where you find tension. Now, when you find this tension, try to feel what's behind it. For example, when you get to your stomach you may find that it feels like a knot, like you're somehow blocked. Maybe you're feeling some jitters about your next prenatal appointment. Or, perhaps you're anxious about how your baby is doing. You might find some happy or sad feelings in the heart area, or you might just feel a warm glow. When you get to your throat area you could feel some tension, like you're trying to say something awkward or embarrassing.

Whenever you locate a feeling, just identify what it feels like and name it something for now: "That sad feeling" or "That nervous feeling." Then, breathe it out, let it go, and keep moving up your body. Just make a note of any inner feelings. Don't worry if you don't find any worries – you may not have any. When you finally get to your head and brain, you may feel that you've got some issues to consider or you may feel clearer already that you've uncovered those issues. Accept whatever feelings you have, move on to steps 7-10 as before, and let yourself become calm and peaceful.

23

Week 7 Objective:
Discover your feelings.

Week 7 & 8 Quiet Time:

Proceed with your normal Quiet Time routine, moving up your body to the next step:

 Track 2

6. When you find tension, ask yourself: What's the feeling here? What's behind the tension? What's really bothering me?

7. Try and label this feeling as either a) emotional worry, or b) an issue that you need do something about now, requiring an action or decision.

8. When you find a feeling that you accept as "normal" then breathe it out and say, "I am letting this go."

9. When you find a feeling that's behind a nagging problem you need to solve, breathe it out and say, "I will solve this soon."

10. When you reach your head and find any remaining or persistent feelings, say, "Calm and peaceful, peaceful and clear" and repeat for one minute. Then return to your regular state, feeling refreshed.

Week 8 Objective:
Learn to accept all your feelings.

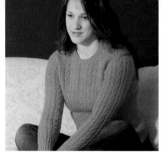

PHOTO: ROGER SALLS

Feelings to Accept/ Feelings to Address

During this stage of your pregnancy, your entire body chemistry is changing to take care of two. If you're like most pregnant moms during the second month, your hormonal changes are making you tired, sometimes nauseated, and maybe also sensitive or moody. You may feel super excited one day, and worried about how you're ever going to handle this the next. These are the natural feelings that you'll probably learn to ACCEPT as part of the flow of your pregnancy. This is also a good time to find someone who's been through pregnancy and childbirth who can share her experiences with you.

Alongside commonplace emotional swings are concerns about practical issues that may require some ACTION. Common problems that occur when bringing a child into the world include relationship issues with your partner, work schedule or career decisions, financial issues, birthing or infant care plans. Whatever the practical problems are, you need to get them out on the table so you can do something about them.

Use Quiet Time to know the difference. This week and next, you'll focus on accepting and letting go of the natural feelings that come with the child-bearing territory and addressing the problems that need a solution or require some assistance.

Perhaps you've heard people say:

"Grant me the serenity to accept the things I cannot change, the courage to change the things I can, and the wisdom to know the difference." This wise attitude may help you to understand and deal with your feelings.

Week 8 Objective:
Create an affirmation to handle feelings.

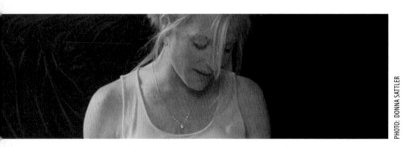

PHOTO: DONNA SATTLER

Say your affirmation out loud each day before you take your Quiet Time and say it out loud in front of the mirror every night before you go to bed and each morning when you get up.

SINCE IT TAKES A WHILE sometimes for feelings or issues to surface, we recommend using your Quiet Time this week to continue to discover, accept, and address any feelings that arise. Toward the end of the week you should be getting a clearer handle on them.

"I am working out the problem with _____

_____ ."

Also, start working this week to create a new affirmation—a promise to yourself how you're going to be and do the best you can—to handle all aspects of your pregnancy. If you've uncovered a strong negative feeling that's simmering behind a pressing problem you need to address, create an affirmation for that. Here are some examples that may help you craft an affirmation that is most meaningful and helpful to you:

"*I am handling* and *addressing my feelings.*"

"*I have a right to my feelings.*"

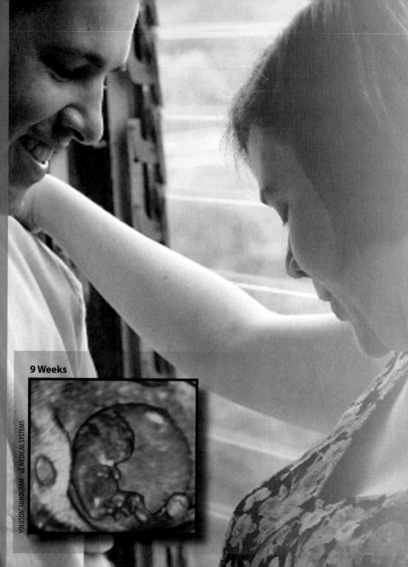

» By nine weeks old your unborn baby is about one inch long and recognizable as human. Baby's eyes, ears, nose and mouth have appeared and hands, fingers, feet and toes can be seen. Your unborn baby moves about freely in the womb, and studies have shown that he or she can respond to touch.

» The unborn baby can kick and bend his head when his nose is touched. By twelve weeks your unborn baby's genitals begin to develop and the baby is recognizable as a boy or girl. Brain development is rapid now and the parts of the brain dealing with behavior and emotions are being laid down.

9 Weeks

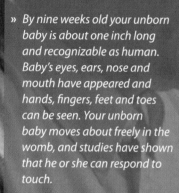

VOLUSON® SONOGRAM - GE MEDICAL SYSTEMS

Month 3 Goal:
Use Quiet Time with your partner to build strength and confidence.

Week 9 Objective:
Understand your role in providing a safe and healthy womb environment.

Relieving stress

Though stress is normal, pregnant women are often reluctant to admit being anxious. Keeping it all inside can make the situation worse. You may feel a pressure to make a perfect baby, or to be a certain kind of mother. You might be a person with too many activities and commitments, and you might have trouble with letting some of them go so you can take care of yourself and your baby.

It can be hard to talk about these things, but it can help to talk to your midwife or doctor, learn calming techniques, or work with a therapist.

Tips for reducing stress:

» Get plenty of rest and sleep.
» Exercise regularly unless you have been advised not to.
» Eat regular meals throughout the day.
» Avoid cigarettes, alcohol, recreational drugs, and caffeinated beverages.
» Scale back work and other commitments.
» Let housework wait or find help with it.
» If high stress persists, talk with your health care provider about it.

Week 10 Objective:
Create an affirmation for growing strong

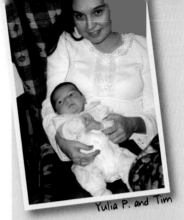
Yulia P. and Tim

My Pregnancy Journal

Write out ways that you could change your lifestyle or attitude to provide a healthier environment for yourself and your baby.

I could help myself and my baby grow stronger if I … _____

_____

I am learning to cope with my pregnancy by… _____

_____

I am gaining greater confidence in myself by… _____

_____

A Parent's Experience

"I guess you have to understand that it's a little person. Even though he's not born yet, he already has a heart and all that kind of stuff. Just understand that it's someone that can't take care of himself. I thought, 'I should pay attention to what I eat and what I do, and if it's going to be good for him or not..' I quit smoking, I didn't smoke at all.

Yulia P. and Tim
– Illinois

Quiet Time
affirmation for Week 10

Use your daily Quiet Time to create your own "Growing Stronger" affirmation—a promise to yourself how you're going to be and do the best you can and repeat it out loud in front of the mirror with conviction each night before and morning after you get out of bed. Some examples: *"I am growing healthier every day" (by eating right or not smoking or drinking), "I am a strong and confident mother."*

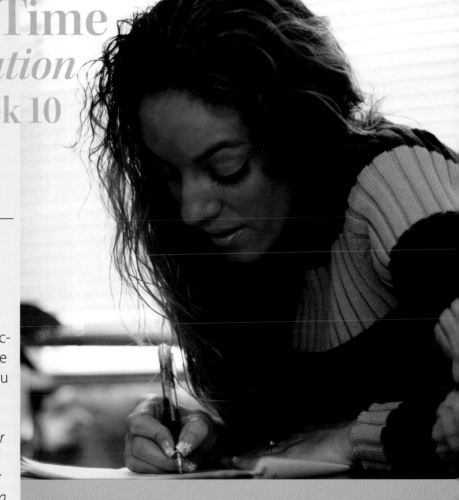

I am: _____

Week 11 Objective:

Involve your partner in your daily Quiet Time.

You're in this together. Up until now you've been learning about your role as mother-to-be and practicing your Quiet Time—right? If you haven't already, it's time to get your partner or a trusted family member or friend to lend their active support.

Start by asking your partner to read page 9 to understand the contribution they can make now to help raise a healthy, happy baby. Then, ask him to complete the Partner's Journal section on pages 111 and 112.

Share what you've learned and share feelings. Start getting your partner involved by sharing what you've been doing so far. Maybe include some of the ideas you've put in your journal and the affirmations you've made. Realize that your partner is facing a lot of changes too and try and get him to share some of his thoughts

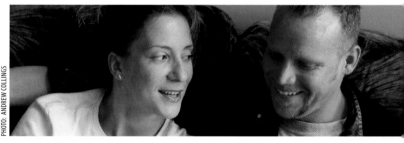

PHOTO: ANDREW COLLINGS

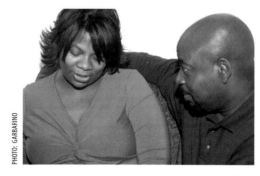

about your new life together. Together, look at your baby's sonogram (if you had one) or the one on page 28 and talk about how far baby has already grown.

Ask for his help. Explain to your partner, friend or family member how important it is for you to keep your stress level down and that he can help in two big ways: 1) by being understanding in his daily relations with you, and 2) by participating in Quiet Time sessions with you. Explain to him how Quiet Time works. Ask him to be the reader and lead you through the 10 steps, or you could talk through it and show him. You might want to tell him that he'll soon be able to experience a little miracle – hearing baby's heartbeat at a prenatal visit.

 Track 1

Do a Quiet Time together. Start by lying down or getting comfortable somewhere together. You can either have your partner play track 1 on the CD or have him slowly read the 10-step Quiet Time on page 16. In either case, when you reach your tummy and you feel comfortable, ask your partner to place his hands with yours over baby and together send thoughts of love to your unborn. If it feels right, you can ask your partner if he wants to kiss the baby or tell her something important.

Week 12 Objective:

Use your daily Quiet Time to find music that relaxes you.

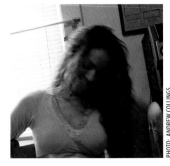

PHOTO: ANDREW COLLINGS

Music is one of the best ways to help the body recover from stress. The right relaxing music can help ease your body and mind, and a calm mother can also mean a calm baby. Later you're going to use music and song to reach and perhaps even entertain your unborn. This week you need to find music that simply soothes YOU.

As you've been taking Quiet Time and listening to the CD, you may have noticed the soft sounds playing in the background. This music was specifically composed and recorded by a top artist in the field to soothe the listener, so you may have already felt the powerful effects of music. This week we want you to fully experience this power and start forming the habit of listening to soothing music throughout the rest of your pregnancy.

Track 3

Your music Quiet Time.
Start by gathering together any relaxing music you may have, or advance your CD player to selection 3 on our CD. Go into your private place and begin to get into a comfortable position. You may want to ask your partner to join you, as it can be easier to have someone else advance the selections while you listen.

1. Get comfortable and take several slow, deep breaths until you feel a natural rhythm of breathing.

2. Close your eyes and take a couple of minutes to focus on your body, starting with your toes. Pause for a moment to feel if you have any tension there, then keep moving up your body, experiencing any tightness in any part. Just notice the tension, and move on.

3. Once you've reached your head and noticed any tension in your face or anxious thoughts in your head, then turn on (or ask your partner to turn on) our CD selection track 3 or your first music selection and see how it makes you feel.

4. Listen to the tune quietly for a minute or two and let the music play over you. Don't think about it with your mind, just experience how the music makes your body feel.

5. Does the music seem to float away tension? Does your body feel more relaxed? Does the melody soothe you?

6. If you found that our music CD really works for you, or your own favorite music soothes you better, just stay with it for a while and let the sounds soothe your body and mind.

7. Come back to this music later in the week or whenever you've had a particularly rough day and need to get away for a while and rejuvenate. Using music throughout your pregnancy can make a big difference to your state of mind.

Month 4 Goal:

Be able to picture my baby in my mind.

Week 13 Objective:

Understand baby's development
and your role in it.

» By the 16th week your baby weighs about 5 ounces and is about 5-6 inches long.

» By week 14 baby's eyes are sensitive to light and can move.

» Baby's brain cells are growing at a rate of 250,000 cells per minute.

» At 14 weeks baby can start making facial expressions including a frown.

» By 14 weeks your unborn can swallow and taste the difference between bitter and sweet.

» By week 15 your baby can hear sounds from outside the womb and may even cover her ears in response to a loud noise.

» By 16 weeks your baby's heart has become fully developed.

» Your baby is moving more, making breathing motions and hiccupping.

» Your fetus is starting to look more like a baby but with a much larger head.

» At this stage, if baby's lips are stroked in the womb, sucking motions are made in response.

» By now baby can kick his feet and curl his toes and may begin sucking his thumb.

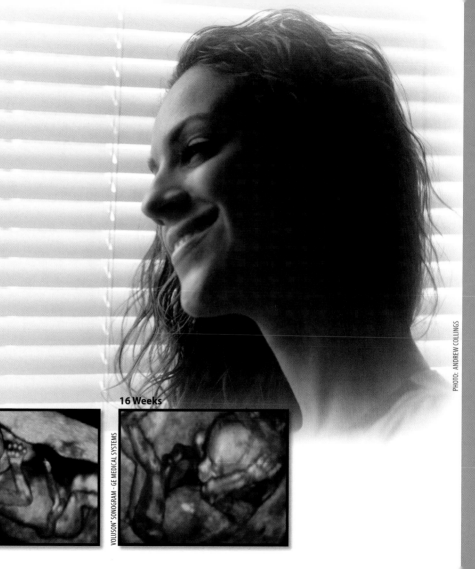

14 Weeks

VOLUSON® SONOGRAM - GE MEDICAL SYSTEMS

16 Weeks

VOLUSON® SONOGRAM - GE MEDICAL SYSTEMS

Week 13 Objective:

Continue to spend your Quiet Time reflecting upon your own baby's development.

Your connection to your unborn

As you can see by typical development at this time, your unborn is experiencing amazing growth and developing remarkable sensitivities in the womb.

If you've been taking Quiet Time on a daily basis you'll probably be feeling more relaxed and alert. This is also helping your baby. Breathing exercises have been shown to reduce your blood pressure, slow down your heart rate and improve your lung function. This helps give you a strong circulation system and a healthy placenta so your baby can best take in oxygen and nutrients and get rid of wastes.

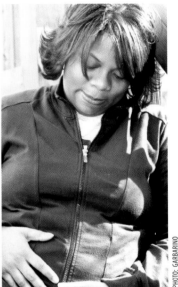

PHOTO: GARBARINO

While we're on the topic of breathing, it's an excellent time to say a bit about chemicals and poisons you may be exposed to. Whether it's something you use or breathe at work, cigarettes you smoke or that your partner smokes, pills and drugs you take while pregnant, alcohol at a cocktail party, or pollution in the air or water, chemicals are a big stress on a pregnant woman and even BIGGER stress on her baby. Chemicals you're in contact with can injure genes in your body or your baby's, and many of them tighten the blood vessels in the placenta, which cuts down the baby's supply of nutrients and oxygen. Most chemicals have unknown effects on growing babies, though we have seen some sad things with chemicals in the past.

Do your baby a favor now and if you smoke, drink alcohol, use recreational drugs or take over the counter medicines—stop! Think about your environment and whether there are chemicals you can do without or avoid. Some things you can't change—but there are many things you CAN do, and even small steps in the right direction will help.

Week 14 Objective:
Think and write about what baby might look like.

My Pregnancy Journal

This is a good time for you and the father or partner to think and make your guesses about what baby might look and be like. But they're just guesses! Your baby will be special and unique in ways you can't imagine yet, and that's part of the joy of parenting. It's also time to start to think about who'll be responsible for what after your baby is born.

I think baby will have: **Partner thinks:**

Eyes like_____   Eyes like_____

Hair like_____   Hair like_____

I'd like a boy or girl or either because:

_____

_____

Your father would like a girl or boy or either because:

_____

_____

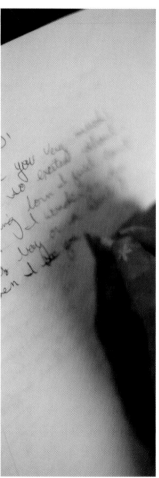

PHOTO: ANDREW COLLINGS

A Parent's Experience

"I was really sensitive when the baby was moving and kicking. Being in tune with that kind of calmed my nerves.... I remember lying down at the end of the day. My day would have quieted and then the nocturnal activity started. I would put my feet up and just sit there and wait for him to get going.... I was imagining if the baby was going to have his color eyes or my color eyes. I was envisioning cradling him in my arms. Then, to touch my stomach and know that there's a little person in there—just to feel connected. It was contact... All of the sudden it starts to come together. This is a life inside of me and that's pretty awesome... I was so ready. I did feel that once he was born, I had always known exactly what he would be like.

Susi C. and Daniel
—New York

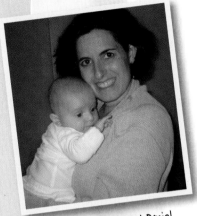

Susi C. and Daniel

I was envisioning cradling him in my arms.

41

I think baby will most look like: _____

Father thinks baby will look most like: _____

I think baby's personality will be: _____

_____

Father thinks baby's personality will be: _____

_____

I'm guessing baby will inherit these kinds of traits from:

_____

_____

Father's guessing baby will inherit these kinds of traits from:

_____

_____

Once you are born I'm really looking forward to doing these kinds of things with you:_____

_____

Father is looking forward to doing these kinds of things with you:

_____

Some of the names we're now considering for our baby are:

If it's a boy:

_____

_____

_____

If it's a girl:

_____

_____

_____

Who is going to take what proportion of responsibilities for baby care?

	Mom %	Dad %
Feeding the baby	_____	_____
Bathing the baby	_____	_____
Tending baby at night	_____	_____
Changing baby	_____	_____

Week 15 Objective:

Use Quiet Time to imagine what your baby might look like.

NOTE: By now, you have probably heard your baby's heartbeat during a prenatal visit. There's a place to record your feelings about that special event on page 50.

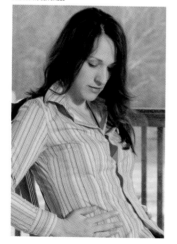

This week and next you're going to use your daily Quiet Time to develop a picture of your baby in your mind. Please note that if these kinds of exercises are not in your cultural, religious or family traditions, you don't need to do them—or maybe you can adapt the concepts to your own beliefs. If you have had a sonogram of your baby and they gave you a picture to take home, you can use it in this exercise. Otherwise, turn to the sonogram pictures on page 37, which give you a pretty good idea of what baby looks like at this stage. Always keep in mind that your baby may not end up looking like you imagined him during these exercises. It is your feelings toward your baby, not an ideal picture, that matter most.

 Track 4

After you've settled into a comfortable position, turn to CD track 4 and follow your pregnancy coach or turn back to page 16 and follow the basic Quiet Time steps. (You can have your partner slowly read each of the steps and pause along the way.) Once you've come to step 6 and reached your growing lower abdomen, we want you to start picturing your baby inside.

Step 7: Picture your baby floating in the warm fluids of your womb, feeling safe, relaxed and content.

8. Notice your baby's tiny toes and his little feet and ankles. See his legs connected to his hips and up to his soft, round tummy.

9. Visualize baby's belly button where the cord connects you to your baby. Feel your love reaching inside your baby. "This is from mommy."

10. Become aware of how safe and relaxed baby is feeling as your love is received. Baby recognizes that this goodness and warmth is coming from you. Take a moment to feel the connection.

11. Now imagine baby's chest, where the heart is beating in a fast and steady rhythm. Become aware of baby's tiny hands and fingers. Look at his growing arms and elbows connecting to his shoulders.

12. Become aware of baby's head. Notice baby's hair, the color that you imagine it to be. Now look at baby's tiny nose, then up to the eyes showing you the color you think they might be.

13. Watch your baby for a moment. Notice how the face seems content and glowing. Feel how your child feels safe and loved. Let your baby know that you will leave your love there to protect him.

14. Begin to say goodbye to baby for now, but continue to feel connected. Then repeat several times: "Feeling connected, connected and loved."

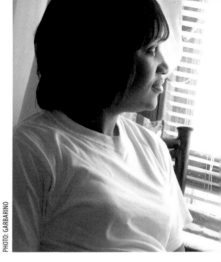

PHOTO: GARBARINO

15. Now slowly take a deep breath and focus on your stomach, slowly breathing in and out for a while. When you are ready, open up your eyes and come back to the room feeling safe and relaxed.

WEEK 16 Objective:
Use your Quiet Time to send growing love to your baby.

Sending love to grow on.
During this exercise of imagining your baby you can also send thoughts and feelings of love to help him grow strong. You can do this exercise alone at first by listening to your Pregnancy Coach on track 5, or ask your partner to join in by reading the steps and guiding you. Or, he can put his hands on your tummy and send his own love to help baby grow. Start by:

6. Picturing your baby floating in the warm fluids of your womb, feeling safe, relaxed and content. Focus on that image for 30 seconds.

7. Take a slow, deep breath and, as this breath reaches your lungs, imagine being filled up with your loving thoughts, glowing warm, soft and soothing.

8. Take another deep breath and as you exhale, send this warm glow of love out of your body and notice how it gently floats above and around both you and your baby. This glow is full of your goodness and love.

9. Now, with another breath, visualize this glow traveling down towards your womb. Let this love enter your body through your belly button and gently swirl into the warm fluids and surround your baby. Feel this love reaching and softly bathing baby.

10. Tell your baby this is from mommy. Stay with the picture of your baby floating with this love and feeling its strength and energy. Then, let baby know you are leaving this love in your womb and that it will help him grow in the months ahead. Tell baby goodbye and with another breath, bring your focus back to the room.

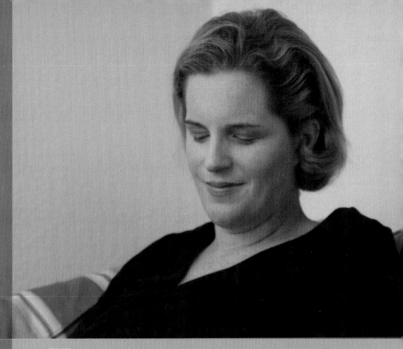

Now, create a new affirmation—a promise to yourself how you're going to do the best you can—to picture your baby in the womb.

Example: "I see my baby growing strong and healthy." Write out your affirmation on the next page and start off each Quiet

I promise

Promise yourself to do the best you can to picture your baby.

My Affirmations

_____

_____

_____

_____

_____

_____

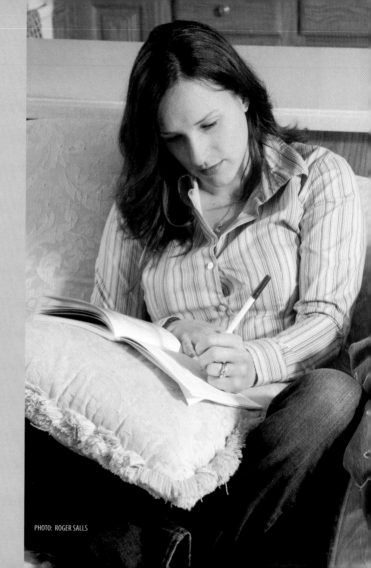

Picturing your baby floating in the warm fluids of your wo...
feeling safe, relaxed and content. Focus on that image for 30 sec...
...ake a slow, deep breath and, as this breath reaches your lungs, ...
...ing filled up with your lo... ...arm, so...
...othing. Take another deep ... ...nd this ...
...glow of love out of your bo... ...ly floats ...
...round both you and your ba... ...your goo...
...ve. Now, with another bre... ...aveling a...
...wards your womb. Let the ... ...ugh you...
...utton and gently swirl into ... ...ound yo...
...eel this love reaching and softly bathing baby. tell your baby t...
...from mommy. Stay with the picture of your baby floating...
...his love and feeling its strength and energy. Then, let baby kno...
...e leaving this love in your womb and that it will help him...
...n the months ahead. Tell baby goodbye and with another brea...

Create your own affirmation for imagining baby.

Month 5 Goal:

To feel and begin to communicate
with my baby.

Week 17 Objective:

Write about your experience and
feelings when you first felt baby move.

Sometime in the next few weeks you'll start to feel your baby move. Women who have been pregnant before usually notice baby movements a little earlier than first time moms do. For many women, feeling baby moving for the first time is an important landmark.

My Pregnancy Journal (continue at the back of the book or in a separate journal)

When I first heard my baby's
heartbeat, I felt_____

_____

_____

The first day I felt my new baby
move was: _____

_____

_____

At the time I was: _____

_____

As a woman, it made me feel_____

_____

The first person I shared this with was: _____

His/her reaction was: _____

_____

How this made me feel about my baby: _____

_____

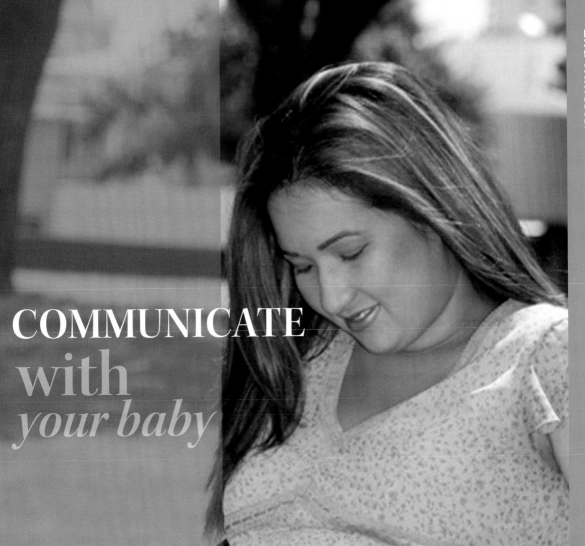

COMMUNICATE
with
your baby

Week 18 Objective:

To understand your unborn baby's development and your role in it.

» Baby is now about 6-8 inches long and weighs one-half pound or more.

» Baby's taste buds are well-developed and baby can taste strong flavors like garlic or curry from mom's diet.

» Baby's hearing apparatus is fully developed by now.

» Baby's brain cells are multiplying at a rate of 50,000-100,000 cells per second.

» By now the connections for feeling pain are in place within the baby's brain.

» Baby's fingerprints are starting to form and her hands can make a firm grip.

» Baby's hiccups can sometimes be seen and felt through your abdomen.

» Baby's nerves between the brain and muscles are developing, allowing her to move in a more coordinated fashion.

18 Weeks

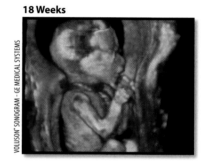

VOLUSON® SONOGRAM - GE MEDICAL SYSTEMS

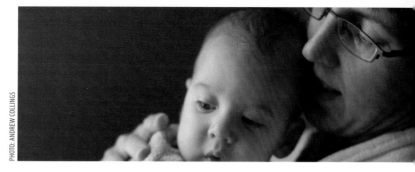

PHOTO: ANDREW COLLINGS

Close in body and mind

Your placenta is now fully developed and your body is becoming more coordinated with that of your unborn. By now your baby is experiencing periods of wakefulness and sleep. Through long hours of watching babies on ultrasound, we are starting to learn about their rhythms and behaviors.

You may begin to notice, as you get more accustomed to your baby's movement, that he has daily patterns or habits – times when you feel like he's awake and active, other times when he's usually quiet, or sleeping. Some babies seem to get active just when you are wanting to settle down for the night. Others have activity patterns that seem very much like your own. Connecting with your baby through these patterns of activity and rest is one way that the two of you are building your relationship together. What can you learn from your baby's habits and responses to what you do? Do you think he might be teaching you something, too?

Gentle Reminder: At your next prenatal visit you can double-check how many weeks along you are, but don't get hung up trying to pin yourself or your baby down on a timeline! Babies grow at different rates and have different personalities. Relax and have fun with your baby!

Week 19 Objective:
Create an affirmation for bonding.

Feeling the parent-child bond

Soon, if you haven't already, you'll feel your baby move inside of you (called "quickening"). For some, this is a miraculous time and fills you up with warm, protective feelings that only a parent can have for a child. For some mothers, it's really cool or maybe even a little scary. Whatever you may be feeling, the reality of pending motherhood is getting, well, very real.

The quickening can also accelerate the bonding process. By bonding we mean the deep feelings –an emotional investment – a mother feels toward and makes in her new baby. You may not feel bonds with your baby until after she or he is born. And those bonds don't appear reciprocal until months after birth – often with baby's first smile or gaze of recognition. So, understand that bonding is a long-term emotional process that proceeds on its own natural course and varies from mom to mom and baby to baby.

The love, caring, and nurturing that comes out of a mother's bond for her baby is as critical to a child's healthy development as is food and safety. So it's not only possible but desirable that a mother-to-be start building bonds early. For many women, the period after quickening inspires them to begin feeling especially protective of their unborn. This is the perfect time to tap into your inner strength and work at empowering yourself to take on your new role as parent.

Creating
YOUR OWN
Bonding *affirmation*

One of the first ways you can start that bonding process is to access your inner spirit and strength through an affirmation that brings out your best. Create your own affirmation and promise yourself you will become the best mother you can be. When you say it, you will feel strong and good.

Say it often with feeling and it will prime you for bonding and psych you up for motherhood. Some examples:

"I am getting closer to you every day."

"I am feeling more and more like a mother."

"I am growing a loving bond with

(If you've chosen a name) _____ my baby"

I am _____

_____

(Say your affirmation aloud before your daily Quiet Time and at the start and end of the day.)

Week 20 Objective:
Begin reaching out to your baby with your own words.

Reaching out to your baby

In the next few weeks we're going to be showing you how you can start communicating with your baby in the womb and get prepared for responsive parenting. Once baby is born, all his senses will be focused on you providing for him. He will be dependent on you to take the lead, and his brain is wired to receive signals from you that teach him how to be a human being. The love and care you express and give to your child is what will make all the difference in his upbringing and happiness.

Start now by reaching into your heart and finding words that capture your feelings toward your baby and express them every day. Some of the best ways to start the communication process is to write a little love letter, story, or poem to your baby. Don't worry if you're not much of a writer; we'll give you ideas and a start. The most important thing is to put yourself into it and write what you care about and want to say. Sharing your feelings through words will help you become closer.

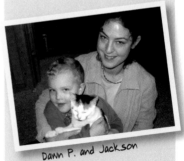

Dawn P. and Jackson

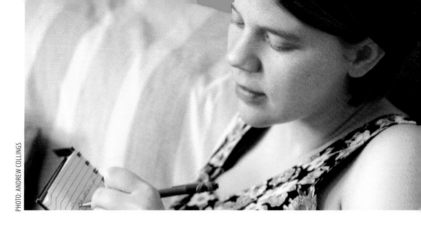

Write a letter. What do you want to tell your baby about you or your new life together? You could introduce yourself and your family, what you do, or where you live. You could tell your child that you're looking forward to meeting him and what you're going to do together after he's born. Tell baby how much love you already have. Start by writing— Dear Baby: I want to tell you...

Write a story. It's simpler than you think. All stories take a journey of some kind where the characters (in this case, your family) face some kind of problem or dilemma (which you can picture as a climb up a hill) and meet a challenge in life (the peak of the hill).

The characters in your story face the challenge (come down the hill) and become the better for it. Think of a simple children's tale like Peter Rabbit. A hungry Peter sneaks into Farmer McGregor's garden to find vegetables, gets caught

and trapped, escapes, and learns a lesson. Believe it or not, even the most long and complex novels are structured the same way. So go ahead, begin your story with a central character, like yourself, and a challenge you're facing. Start climbing the hill!

Write a poem. You don't have to be a poet. It doesn't have to rhyme or be long. Concentrate on your feelings and your hopes for baby. It can be as little as the way you've decorated the nursery to as lofty as imagining the first time you'll see his face. Just start by creating a title that captures a way you are feeling, start the first line and let it flow.

You can use the back pages of this book or a separate journal for your writing. Then read your poem, letter or book every day to baby this week and next.

Children's books. Besides writing and sharing something personal, reading is one of the best ways to connect with your unborn. Go to your library or bookstore and get a collection of nursery rhymes or a Dr. Seuss book you like and read one every night before bed. The simple words and repetition are like a playground song or a lullaby. And by reading to your baby on a regular basis, you will be forming a habit that, if continued, will help prepare your child for school success.

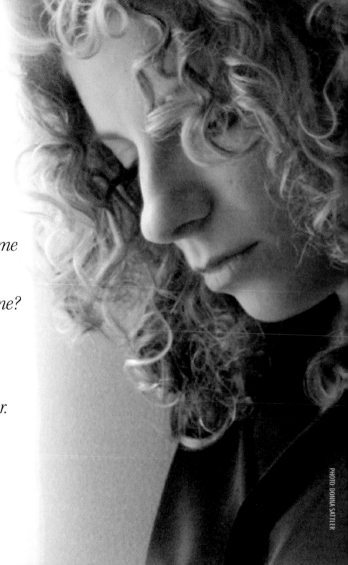

Here's what one mom wrote to her baby:

I'm right here, baby,
Let's hold tight.
They say my life won't be the same
Won't be like before you came.
But, baby, baby what's your name?

I'm right here baby,
Friend and mother.
Our bond won't be like any other.
Together we will both discover
How to make a family.
Baby, baby, you and me.

Month 6 Goal:
Communicating with my baby.

Week 21 Objective:
Understand your unborn baby's development and your role in it.

» Baby is now about 7-9 inches long and weighs nearly a pound.

» By 22 weeks a baby can respond to touch and sound and react to loud noises (which can even cause a jumping reaction).

» Brain parts that control conscious thought are starting to develop now.

» By now, baby begins to have definite sleep and wakeful periods.

» Right about now the buds for baby's permanent teeth will come in.

» The smallest blood vessels of baby's body—the capillaries—are starting to grow and give baby's skin a pinkish glow.

21 Weeks

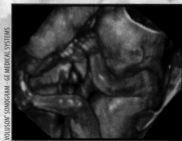

VOLUSON® SONOGRAM - GE MEDICAL SYSTEMS

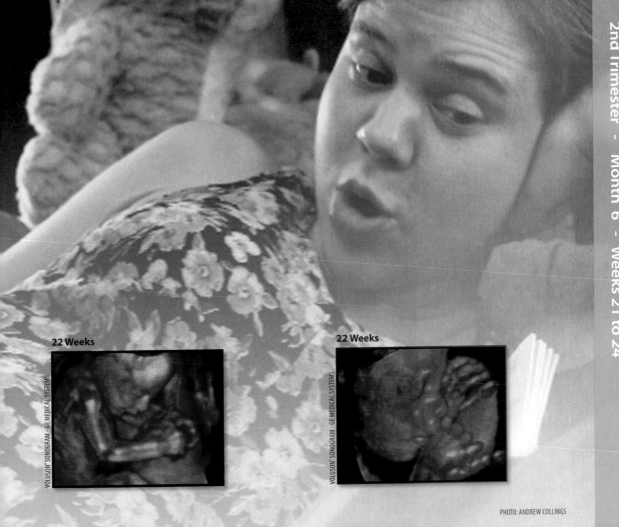

22 Weeks

22 Weeks

VOLUSON® SONOGRAM - GE MEDICAL SYSTEMS

VOLUSON® SONOGRAM - GE MEDICAL SYSTEMS

Week 21 Objective:

Understanding communication between you and baby

Hearing, remembering and liking your voice

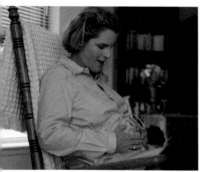

PHOTO: ALAN LEMIRE

Out-loud conversations between a mother and her unborn baby may lay the foundations of communication after birth, as well as increase the mother-infant bond. Also, research is beginning to show that babies can learn and perhaps even remember what was heard in the womb! (Not words, of course, but the rhythms of language.)

Hearing is one of the strongest senses for babies before they are born. For instance, an unborn not only hears and recognizes the sounds of his mother's voice in the womb, but based on fetal heart rate patterns, scientists believe he is also calmed by it. Unborn babies remember the sound of their mother's voice from the womb and once born, seem to show a preference for listening to their mother's voice over other females. Babies also seem to be able to recognize rhymes. One study showed that when mothers repeated a certain children's rhyme daily from week 33 to 37, later on their babies reacted to the rhyme by way of an increased heart rate, but showed no reaction to an unfamiliar rhyme.

Unborn babies begin to learn the tempos and rhythms of their native language and again, based on their nipple sucking response, seem to "prefer" their mother tongue to others they heard.

It was just the two of us.

Babies also seem to prefer to hear stories that were read to them in the womb. Researchers at the University of North Carolina had pregnant mothers read Dr. Seuss's *Cat in the Hat* twice a day to their unborn babies. After birth, they were read another Dr. Seuss book. Based on their nipple sucking response, they remembered The Cat in the Hat story and not the other one, and preferred it when it was read forward, not backwards.

Krista K. and Bridget

A Parent's Experience:

"I never had any negative feelings about being a single mom. I felt like we were going on this journey together. It was just the two of us... I talked out loud a lot because I was by myself a lot... I didn't talk to her about anything profound. It would be more like, 'What shirt should I wear today'?' or, "Now, we're going here or there', just like she was anyone else... After I found out she was a girl, I always addressed her as Bridget... I really felt like she was part of me, but that she was her own person and deserved her own respect."

Krista K. and Bridget
—California

Learn to "listen" to baby's movements.

Communicating by feel

Once baby is born, one of your biggest challenges as a parent will be to understand the meaning of baby's body language and different cries.

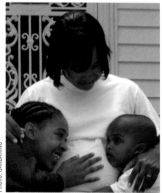

PHOTO: GARBARINO

You will quickly sense and learn what your baby's needs are. Through trial and error, you'll come to know the difference between a cry of hunger and a cry caused by gas. Being attuned to your child's feedback to your actions is also a central part of parenting. Just like in any other relationship, sensitive, two-way communication between you allows you to work together effectively as a team.

You can start now.

What's amazing is that you can start learning lessons in responsive parenting right now. Every day, get in the habit of tuning in to baby's thumps and bumps in the womb. Many of these movements are the reflexive kind, which are essential to a baby's motor development and survival after birth. However, some movements can be in response to what's going on outside the womb. Very soon you will be able to communicate with your baby through your voice and touch. Your baby just may "talk" back to you through movement.

All you have to do is become aware of and sensitive to your child's varying movements, and practice the exercises.

My Pregnancy Journal

"Listening" for baby's movements is the starting point for your "conversations." For the next few weeks, use these journal questions to record your baby's movements:

When is baby most active?

_____

Does baby move around inside in different ways? (fast, slow, etc.)

_____

_____

Does baby ever move in a certain way when you do something?

_____

How does it feel when baby moves?

_____

_____

(Continue your journal of baby's movement patterns on page 110.)

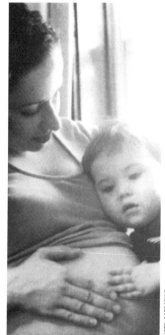

PHOTO: GARBARINO

Learn to talk with baby

Quiet Time for talking.

This week we're going to ask you to begin, if you haven't already, talking <u>with</u> your baby. Even though your baby cannot talk back, your voice can be heard. By asking your baby questions and thinking about what he or she might be feeling, you are learning to become a responsive parent. During this Quiet Time, you'll be asked to picture yourself holding and playing with your baby and imagining your child's reactions. With time and practice, you may be able to feel baby responding to your words, tone of voice, and feelings. First, begin to believe that you can. Then empower yourself to begin talking with your baby by creating your own affirmation.

Examples:
"I am able to communicate with you now." "I am talking with baby and she is hearing me."

I am: _____

_____

_____

_____

_____

_____

_____

_____

_____

_____

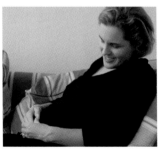

PHOTO: ALAN LEMIRE

Track 6

To begin, ask your partner to stay around for a while to join you in a Quiet Time with baby. Then, when you feel baby becoming active, take 15 minutes together. Go into a quiet room and get into a comfortable position and play CD track 6, or ask your partner to slowly read the paragraphs below while you close your eyes and begin to picture your baby. As you partner reads, imagine that you are communicating with baby.

"Hello, little baby, how are you?

This is your mommy (daddy) *speaking.*

Are you nice and warm inside where you are?

Each day you are getting bigger, and when you are big enough and ready, you will be born.

I can hardly wait. I hope you like all the good foods we are eating and that you are growing healthy and strong."

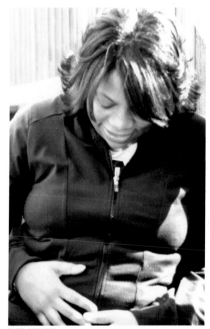

PHOTO: GARBARINO

Use your Quiet Time to practice talking with baby.

Note: Remember to first tell baby who's speaking. Speak loudly, and always pause after a question to listen and feel for a response.

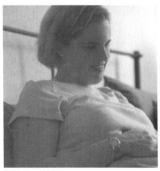

PHOTO: ALAN LEMIRE

"How are you feeling today?" (pause and listen for what your baby might say)

"Can you hear me talking?" (pause)

"What are you doing in there now?" (pause)

"Are you awake or resting?" (pause)

"Are you sucking your thumb?" (pause)

"Are you stretching?" (pause)

"I can hardly wait until you are born – when I can see your face and you recognize me."

"I think about holding you and calling your name. I can see myself rubbing and kissing your soft head. Won't that feel good?"

"How about when I tickle your tummy? Will you kick your legs and giggle?"

"I can see myself patting your little behind. Will that make you laugh?"

"Are you getting excited, too, about playing with me?"

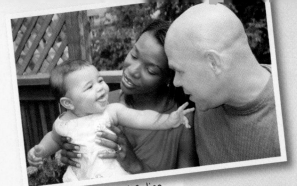

Jonathan H., Ebele and Celice

"Soon baby, we will be having great fun together, but now it is time for you to rest."

"Do you feel tired now? Are your eyes starting to close?"

It's time to say goodbye now, baby, so you can have a nice sleep. We can talk and play another day. Stay safe and warm."

NOW OPEN YOUR EYES AND SLOWLY COME BACK TO THE ROOM.

I'd get right up there and talk to my daughter in her mother's belly...

A Parent's Experience:
"I'd get right up there and talk to my daughter in her mother's belly, I primarily talked to her about dating. I tried to plant in her head that dating is unacceptable until age 26, so I'm hoping that sticks. We also talked about her credit report and how important that is, along with other financial issues, the markets — when not to invest."

Ebele, Jonathan H. and Celice
—Illinois

69

Talk with your baby every day.

How you and baby can benefit from daily conversation:

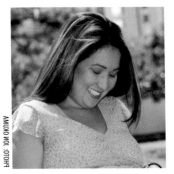

PHOTO: JON OKUMA

» Listening to your baby with undivided attention will ready you and make you feel good about being responsive after birth.

» By talking with your unborn baby, you can prepare yourself for accepting your baby and start to develop bonds of affection.

» The positive communication habits you develop now will last throughout life.

» Talking with your baby in the womb will create a link between your voice patterns and baby's reactions. Your child may become more attentive to you after birth.

Create your greeting for baby:
Each day when you meet people, say at work or in a store, it's common courtesy that you first acknowledge them with a polite, "Hello" or "How are you doing?" From now on, do the same with baby each time you feel movement during the day. Create your own natural greeting for baby before you converse. For example: "Well, hello in there –what's my baby doing?" "Hi, baby –how's it going?" "Good Morning, [-name-], how are you today?"

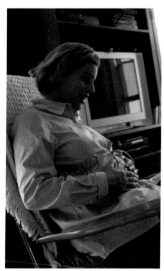

PHOTO: ALAN LEMIRE

Sharing daily conversations.
Once baby is born, you'll be spending a lot of time together talking. This baby talk, also known as "parentese", is very important to a child's learning and language development, and also seems to help your newborn feel safe and secure. Practice parentese now by bringing baby into your every-day routines and activities as through he or she is already a participating member of the family. Talk out loud to baby whenever you feel like it. (Don't be embarrassed: pregnant women do this all the time.) You'll find that baby is a good listener and makes great company.

Have a conversation with baby...

» whenever you think about baby, then tell him/her what you're thinking about.

» whenever you're doing some-thing to get ready for baby, like going shopping or to prenatal visits. Then tell baby about what happened.

» whenever you think about how things are going to be when he/she comes. Tell baby about all the fun you're going to have.

"It's our song, baby."

Month 7 Goal:
Play music for and sing to baby.

Week 25 Objective:
Understand your unborn baby's development and your role in it.

26 Weeks

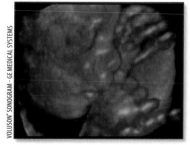

VOLUSON SONOGRAM - GE MEDICAL SYSTEMS

» Baby is now about 10 to 12 inches long and weighs about 2 lbs.

» By the 26th week your baby's lungs are capable of breathing air.

» By the 25th week, baby's brain wave patterns are similar to a full-term baby's at birth.

» By 27 weeks, baby's eyelids begin to part; eyes become sensitive to light and dark.

» Baby's brain continues to grow rapidly and the part of the brain that allows baby to communicate is forming.

» Baby is becoming more responsive to sounds.

» By the 28th week all baby's reflexes that will be evident at birth are present, including sucking, grasping, and stepping.

» By the 28th week, baby will respond by changing facial expressions when he tastes sour or sweet.

» At this age, an unborn can move in rhythm to music.

Week 25 Objective:
Add music to your world together

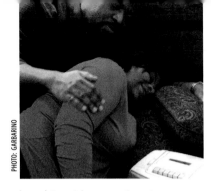

By now your unborn's hearing is fully formed. Your baby can hear your heart beat, voices from outside, and sounds of fluid in her watery world. Some studies suggest that babies may move in the womb to the sound of music, and that lullabies and children's songs may even have a calming effect.

Baby researchers are doing some pretty interesting studies with unborn babies. For instance, they compared a group of pregnant women who watched a soap opera with certain theme music every day with a non-watching group. After birth, the babies who had heard the theme music in the womb reacted distinctly to it, while the other babies did not. Do you think the reaction was directly to the music, or perhaps from the babies' remembering that when the music played, their mothers sat down to relax and watch a show they liked?

Other babies who were exposed to music in the womb will turn their heads toward the familiar sounds and/or change their facial expressions, even seeming to smile, after they are born. Also, they increase their suckling, stretch their fingers and toes, and have a slower heart rate and more regular breathing. It's easy to imagine that these are signals of enjoyment, though impossible to know for sure.

Some researchers believe that babies who "listen to music" before they are born do better on some measures of development while they are infants. Other researchers think this isn't the case. So little is known about what babies can "think" or "learn"! But pretty much everyone agrees that listening to music together with your baby is fun and pleasurable – so give it a try and see what happens.

(To learn more, see the Resources section at the back of the book.)

It's a bond I don't think we'll ever break.

A Parent's Experience

"During my pregnancy I would often sing. It soon became evident that my unborn son preferred some songs and types of music over others. While I was singing certain songs, he would kick vigorously, and during others he would swim around to the beat of the music, a motion I later called 'dancing.' It got to where we had a routine established. If I was practicing for church, every day I would sing particular songs in a certain order, and sure enough, he would move the same way to the same songs every time. Two songs were particularly

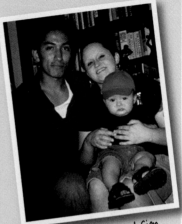

Antonio, Aimee D. and Gian

special. One was a folk song where I substituted my son's name, Gian, where another word would normally go. Now that he's born, when I sing "our" songs, he exhibits the same behavior...excited for some songs, pacified by others. It's a bond I don't think we'll ever break."

Antonio, Aimee D. and Gian
—Texas

Find some relaxing music for you and your baby.

NOTE: By this time many moms (and dads) are already taking childbirth classes, so you might want to review some exercises dealing with labor and delivery – you'll find them in the section on Weeks 33 to Birth, starting on page 92.

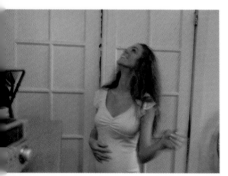

PHOTO: ANDREW COLLINGS

The benefits of music and song: Although you may not even be able to carry a tune, it's a good bet you like listening to some kind of music. Because your unborn baby's brain is now capable of processing sounds, you may be wondering whether music can be pleasing to her, too!

Some moms have said that when they played the same music during labor that they had played before baby was born, they felt as though their babies were more comfortable and secure. Do you think that's possible?

Classical music may not be the kind that relaxes you, but some studies have shown that classical music may be particularly enjoyable for your unborn. Certain baroque music by Bach, Mozart, and Handel moves to the tempo of 60-70 beats per minute – the same rate baby hears from your heart. The selection for week 26 on track 7 on the CD was specially composed to soothe you and baby. If you have some other music like lullabies for a nursery that you enjoy, that's good too.

Week 26 Objective:

Use your daily Quiet Time to select music that relaxes both of you.

Back in week 12 you hopefully found some music that really relaxes you, or you've come to play our CD often to soothe you. This week you'll find and listen to music that soothes both of you and becomes "your tune" that you share together often.

 Track 7

Set-up for your musical Quiet Time.

Start your session by bringing your CD player, our CD, and any other music into your quiet room. You might want to ask your partner to join you as it may be easier for him to play the various tunes while you listen. Place the player near your abdomen where baby can hear and you can reach the controls and adjust the volume to a moderate level.

CAUTION: Don't place headphones on your abdomen; it could be too loud for your baby's delicate ears!

1. Get comfortable and start to take several slow deep breaths until you feel a natural rhythm of breathing.

2. Close your eyes and take a couple of minutes to focus on your body, starting with your toes. Pause for a moment to feel if you have any tension there, then keep moving up your body experiencing any tightness in any part. Just notice the tension and move on.

3. Once you've reached your head and noticed any tension in your face or anxious thoughts in your head, then either you or your partner can turn the CD on to track 7.

4. Listen to the tune quietly for a minute or two and let the music play over you. Don't think about it with your mind, just experience how the music makes your body feel. Does the music seem to float away tension? Does your body feel more relaxed? Does the melody soothe you?

5. If you found that this music feels right for you and baby, then go to the next step on the next page. Or, play some other music selections and see how that feels.

Week 27 Objective:

Use Quiet Time to play music that relaxes both of you.

Now you're going to play your tune to see if baby enjoys it too. Of course, baby hasn't developed her musical tastes yet, so it'll be up to you to sense her reactions.

6. From that relaxed state with the music still playing, focus your attention on your abdomen.

7. Start to picture your baby now lying there in your womb. Notice her tiny toes and growing legs. See the arms and hands floating lazily. When you get to baby's face, say hello and say that you've got a surprise.

8. 8. Tell baby you've got some special music for him/her to listen to. Let it play for a moment, then ask your baby: Do you hear that, baby? It's music. Do you like it? (Pause to listen and feel.) How does this music sound to you, baby?

9. Just listen to the music for a while and wait for any reaction you may get from baby. Do you feel any movement?

10. After a moment, turn the music off and feel if there is any reaction the music being stopped. After a while, put the music back on again or select another tune to see if you get any reaction. If not, try it again later.

NOTE: If you don't sense any reaction, don't worry! It may take time, and not all babies respond to musical sounds anyway. Your baby might be sleeping. You could try to play your tunes when baby is especially active to see if it soothes her. Some babies don't react, but still hear. Music that makes you feel good and relaxed probably makes baby feel good, too!

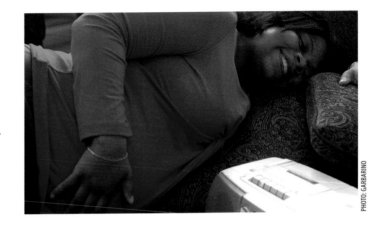

When I played _____ today,

baby responded by_____

_____

I have chosen _____
for our tune and we'll listen to it together once a week, right through labor and delivery.

Week 28 Objective:
Create and sing your own lullaby to baby.

This week you're going to introduce a new instrument into your musical repertoire —your voice. Your talking voice is already your unborn baby's favorite sound, along with your heartbeat. Now you can add melodic interest and soothing rhythms for enjoyment and learning. The quality of your singing doesn't matter to baby, who will just love to feel the vibrations of your diaphragm and hear notes that tickle his ears when you sing.

One of the best ways to connect with baby through song is to create a little lullaby or nursery rhyme that you can perform. It's easy. Don't be surprised if you find that if you sing it regularly while you're pregnant, baby will recognize it after birth and it will have a powerful soothing effect. Here's how:

1. Think of a familiar lullaby you may have heard as a child, like "Twinkle, Twinkle."

2. Hum the tune to yourself as you begin to think of your baby.

3. Write down whatever words or phrases come to mind, including baby's name if you know it. You will probably change the words many times over a few days as you sing your special song.

4. If you'd rather not create your own, just pick one of the lullabies here, or turn to page 113 in the back to find another lullaby or song that you like.

5. Sing it once a day to baby, and invite your partner and family to sing it to your tummy, too! What a nice way to get ready to go to sleep.

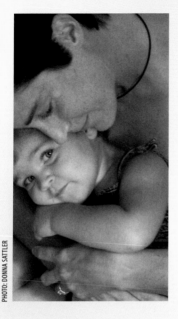

PHOTO: DONNA SATTLER

Twinkle, twinkle, little star (baby's name)
How I wonder what you are.
Up above the world so high,
Like a diamond in the sky.

Hush, little baby (name), don't say a word,
Papa's going to buy you a mockingbird.
If that mockingbird won't sing
Papa's going to buy you a diamond ring.

Mary (Name) had a little lamb
Its fleece as white as snow
And everywhere that _____ went
That lamb was sure to go.

Duérmete, mi niña, (nombre)
duérmete, mi sol,
duérmete, pedazo
De mi corazón.

Twinkle, twinkle, little star

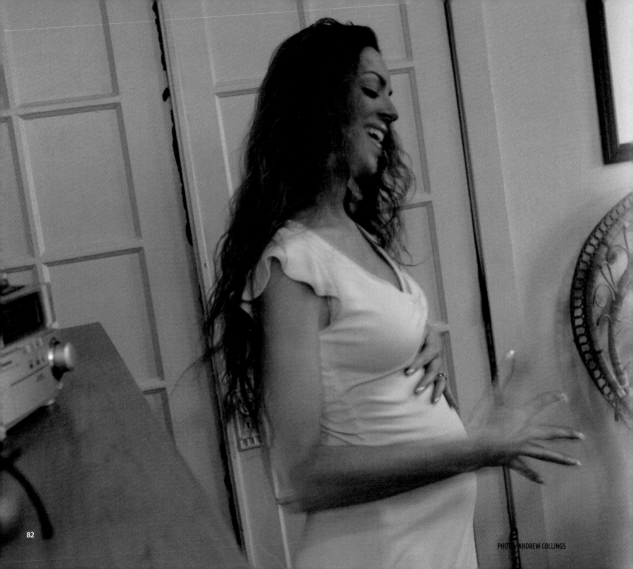

82

Month 8 Goal:
Communicate with baby through movement and touch.

Week 29 Objective:
Learn about baby's development and your role in it.

31 Weeks

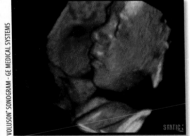

VOLUSON® SONOGRAM - GE MEDICAL SYSTEMS

32 Weeks

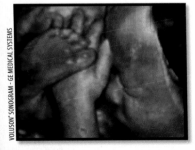

VOLUSON® SONOGRAM - GE MEDICAL SYSTEMS

» By 32 weeks, baby could be around 15 inches long and weigh around 4-5 pounds.

» By 32 weeks, baby's eyebrows and head hair appear.

» By now, your baby may have turned upside down and maybe back again.

» Baby has assumed the fetal position with his legs drawn into his chest because there isn't enough room to stretch out.

» By now, baby is perfectly formed and will be putting on baby fat.

» By 32 weeks, baby's arm and leg muscles are fully linked to his nervous system so that relatively coordinated movement can occur.

» By 32 weeks, baby hears and reacts differently to voices of her mother, father, and others.

» By now, baby's fingernails may have reached the end of his fingertips. As a result some babies may have already scratched their faces in the womb.

» From 32 weeks on, your baby has the maturity to adapt to living outside the womb when born.

Learn about baby's development and your role in it.

Talking with Touch

Have you noticed how much it can help sometimes to feel a hug or a reassuring hand on your shoulder? Touch is a powerful communicator. The womb provides baby with a world of touch, which is thought to be important to early brain development and ultimately, emotional security. From the gentle swirl of amniotic fluid to the tactile sensation of touching the uterine wall whenever you turn, sit, walk or bend, your unborn is sensing you.

Since the 1980s several studies have been conducted on prenatal stimulation. In one program, called the Prenatal University, founded by California obstetrician Dr. Rene Van de Carr, parents were taught to interact with their babies through talk, song, and touch, and by playing a "kick game." Dr. Van de Carr believes that participating families were more pleased with their pregnancy and birth experiences, had a greater parent-to-child bond, and had more confidence in meeting baby's needs. (See the Resources section for more information.)

A program in Thailand, which was similar to the California program, also suggested that infants gained from prenatal enrichment. These babies smiled more, showed better movement skills, talked earlier, and were able to calm themselves more quickly when rocked or patted than babies who hadn't been in the program.

It's hard to study babies in the womb, as you can imagine! More research is needed about fetal learning and development. Still, these early results are fascinating, don't you think?

"Could this tiny life be responding to me?"

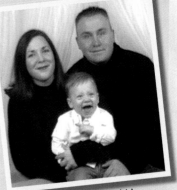

Christie, Tim A. and Aiden

A Parent's Experience

"OK baby, let's take a nap." I lay down and put my hands on the bulge, as I had done so many times before, and closed my eyes for a little rest. Did I feel something? I giggled. Again, a little tickle. The tiny tickle made me laugh out loud. The laugh caused another flutter. Could this tiny life be responding to me? I push back on my belly where he kicked and he would kick back. Were my poking fingers disrupting his world? My laughter disrupting his slumber? Or did this tiny person already have my sense of humor? I knew beyond science or reason that this life, an extension of my own, shared my delight in all things funny. And, I've been laughing with him ever since!

Christie, Tim A. and Aiden
—Oregon

85

Week 30 Objective:
Use Quiet Time to do daily baby massage

Touch is a very important and easy way to communicate emotional security to babies, born or yet to be born.

Whether it's the security of your womb, the soothing stroke of your hand, or the cradle of your arms, babies need to feel your love. The instinct for touch is what makes the bond between parent and child real. Aren't you looking forward to putting your arms around your baby and holding her close? Since your unborn can now sense your touch and may also respond to it, prenatal massage techniques can be an ideal way to build those bonds. Although you'll focus your attention on the palm of your hand and baby's response, feel free to talk or sing with baby during this exercise.

 Track 8

Start by playing track 8 on our CD or have your partner read the steps to you.

1. Take a comfortable position, close your eyes, and relax. Take several long, deep breaths, and once you feel relaxed move to step 2.

2. Place your hands gently over your abdomen. Visualize the shape of your baby's body under your hands. Is baby resting or active?

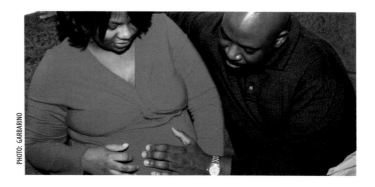

3. Begin to slowly stroke your abdomen from below your belly button to below your breasts using long, broad strokes or circular strokes.

4. As you continue stroking, imagine a warm glow coming from your hands, which expresses your love for your baby. This warm light reaches your baby and touches baby's soft head, back, shoulders, arms, and hands. Then lightly touch the little chest and tummy, legs and feet. Feel the love you have for baby radiating through your hands.

5. Continue stroking. If you sense baby moving around, feel how your baby relaxes as you stroke him or her. Imagine that your baby senses your love and feels safe and secure.

6. Slow the strokes of the massage, but continue to hold your hands on the abdomen for a while until you are ready to open your eyes.

Later, you may find this gentle massage to be very soothing to you while you're in labor. Or maybe you can use this technique to put some nice lotion on your growing belly – how lovely!

Week 31 Objective:
Use Quiet Time to dance with your baby.

In a couple of short months, you'll be able to pick baby up in your arms and dance with him around the room. Since your unborn now hears (and perhaps enjoys) music, why not take the lead and give a few dance lessons?

Think of it: your unborn already senses you walking, exercising, and bouncing around in a car. So imagine how good it might feel to hear music, feel the vibrations of your voice, and experience the gentle sway of your dancing body!

Dancing with baby can be one of the most enjoyable and relaxing ways to build a relationship with your baby.

Get ready to play track 9 on our CD or find some other lively music that makes you feel like dancing. Take your CD player into your Quiet Time space and sit in a comfortable chair and follow the steps below:

 Track 9

1. Put on our CD selection for dancing (or another dance tune you like) and listen to the music for a while, letting it play over your body.

2. Become aware of the music's effect on both your spirit and body. Does it uplift your spirit and make you feel happy? Does it make you start tapping your fingers or toes, or bop your head to the rhythm?

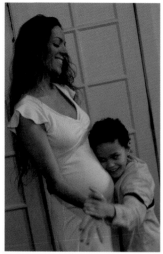

3. Once you find a tune that energizes your body and spirit and makes you feel like dancing, close your eyes and picture and feel baby in your womb. What is baby doing now? Ask if your child can hear and feel the music. Wait for a response. If you and baby feel like it, then ask, "Do you wanna dance?"

4. Stand up and place one or both of your arms around your tummy and begin to sway or dance with the beat of the music. Singing or humming along will make it even more fun.

5. After you've enjoyed one or two songs together, turn the music off, sit or lie down, and listen and feel for baby. Did baby stop dancing or is there still some bopping going on?

6. Ask if baby enjoyed that dance. Listen. Do you sense your little dancer wants another, or that she wants to rest for now? Depending on baby's response and how you feel, take another turn or let your baby have her nap.

NOTES: Check with your health care provider for any precautions about this exercise. Dancing too vigorously is not recommended: use your good judgment. Ask your partner or a sibling if he'd like to join you and baby for the next dance. Just not a dancer? A rocking chair might work for you.

Week 32 Objective:

Use Quiet Time to learn and play the Kick Game

By now you may already be sensing that you're communicating with baby through touch. This week and through the rest of your pregnancy, you can play a little game each time you feel your baby move. The Kick Game is fun!

Playing the Kick Game: The basic idea behind the Kick Game is to teach baby that when he kicks, there will be a response, and that this back and forth interaction is associated with certain sounds. Try to respond consistently to baby's movement as though you were talking with someone.

CAUTION: Do not play this game too often or too vigorously –it could over-stimulate your baby. A gentle few minutes on each occasion is all you need. Remember – most of the day your baby needs to sleep!

Whenever you feel baby is active and you have a few minutes to devote to Quiet Time, then you and baby can proceed to play the Kick Game. Start by putting on track 10 on our CD. With practice you will be able to follow these steps each time you feel like playing.

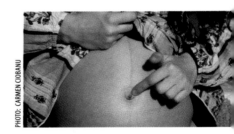

PHOTO: CARMEN CIOBANU

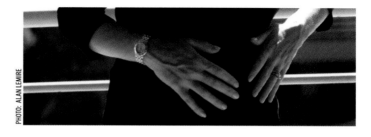

Track 10

Step 1: Gently pat or press your abdomen with one hand where the baby is kicking. Do this for one week, getting used to responding to baby's movements.

Step 2: Locate a paper tube or roll up a large piece of paper into a megaphone shape. During the second week, begin saying the words "kick, kick, kick," speaking through the "megaphone" at the same time you are patting back.

Step 3: If baby starts to kick back where you have been patting your abdomen, you can press back again and you will be "talking" to your baby. Say, "Hi baby, this is mama. Kick. That's a good baby. Kick here again." Be patient—this may not happen right away. (And some babies don't want to play this game at all!)

VARIATIONS: You could also try gently pushing on one side of your tummy, wait, and try pushing on the other side to see if baby "follows" you. Or, try patting your abdomen twice and wait –sometimes babies will kick back twice!

* NOTE: Partners and others can participate too. Have your helper place his cheek on the abdomen with his mouth close to the baby's head. When you feel baby kicking, point to the area and ask him to say, "Hi, this is Daddy. Kick here. That's a good baby. Kick, kick, kick again." Then gently pat the baby's feet.

Month 9 Goal:
Prepare mentally for labor and welcoming baby.

Week 33 Objective:
Understand baby's development and your role in it.

Preparing for Labor

Every woman is a little anxious about giving birth – that's normal and healthy. A high level of fear and stress, however, can put a heavy burden on you and your baby and can even make labor harder. Participation in childbirth classes can prepare you for what to expect and will give you helpful skills for labor. Getting any fears out in the open, discussing them, and finding help can also be beneficial. Relaxation exercises can increase your confidence and self-control and visualizing can make for a more successful labor and birth. Remember that women have been giving birth for a very long time, and your body knows exactly what to do.

If you discover that you have a lot of fears, try to get them out in the open, discuss them with your partner or prenatal care provider, and get help if needed. Use your daily Quiet Time this week to uncover any big worries and create an affirmation to help you handle them effectively.

» In the last weeks of pregnancy, all baby's parts and organs have formed and she is working on growing bigger, filling out and gaining weight. By week 36, the average baby weighs about 6 lbs.

» By 35 weeks, baby's eyes are sensitive to changes in light outside the womb and can blink.

» By now, baby's reflexes and coordination are well established and she's ready to enter the world.

» By now, baby's movements tend to decrease as she has little room in the womb.

» By 37 weeks your baby is considered full-term.

34 Weeks

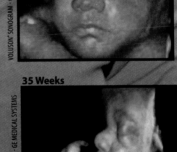

VOLUSON® SONOGRAM - GE MEDICAL SYSTEMS

35 Weeks

VOLUSON® SONOGRAM - GE MEDICAL SYSTEMS

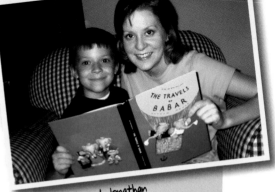
Amy C. and Jonathan

Week 33 Objective:
Uncover your feelings about labor and birth.

He was not just a baby; he was a person.

A Parent's Experience

"As Jonathan was being delivered, the doctor told me, 'Get ready to say 'Happy Birthday to Jonathan.' I'll never forget that. He was not just a baby; he was a person. After he was born, Jonathan knew that he was wanted and loved. As I held him, he was very peaceful and relaxed. There was a sense of recognition when I talked to him. He seemed to say, 'I know who you are: you're my mommy.'"

Amy C. and Jonathan
—Texas

My Pregnancy Journal

Look inward to uncover your true feelings and get them out in your journal. For instance ask:

Do I feel prepared for labor? _____

_____

Do I worry about pain? _____

_____

Do I worry that I might lose control? _____

_____

Do I worry about any complications? _____

_____

The thing that I worry most about is: _____

_____

I want to talk to my midwife or doctor about: _____

_____

I would have greater confidence in my ability to handle labor if I:

_____

Create an affirmation for handling labor. If you've uncovered any fears or unresolved worries, empower yourself to handle them. Create a statement that when spoken will give you the courage and strength to be able to deal with it. Examples: "I am ready and able to handle labor. I can get the information I need. I can trust my body to give birth.

"I am _____

_____

_____

_____

_____

_____

_____

(Say your affirmation in front of the mirror every night before bed and again in the morning)

Use Quiet Time to build confidence for giving birth.

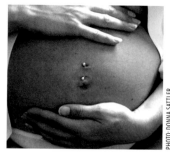

PHOTO: DONNA SATTLER

Track 11

Your baby's birth day may unfold in ways that you cannot plan for or expect. One of the best things you can do for yourself is to stay flexible, calm and confident that you will be mentally ready for whatever happens. This week you'll use your Quiet Time to prepare mentally for labor and birth. Go into your Quiet Place, get comfortable, and turn on the CD to selection 11. Or, ask your partner to slowly read each of the scenes below and pause in between while you imagine yourself facing the big day with ease and confidence.

START by closing your eyes, and begin to breathe deeply and slowly. Feel your body relaxing, and with each breath let go of any tension you feel in your body. Let your body go limp and sink into your chair or bed. Let go of any thoughts in your mind except for the scenes of your baby's birth day. You are about to watch a movie where you'll see yourself performing like a star.

(Read each scene, slowly pausing in between to let mom's mind fully picture and experience the scene).

1. First, picture your planned labor and birth location now in your mind. Everything looks familiar and comfortable to you as you remember it. This is the place where you will first meet your baby. Feel that it is a safe and secure place where everything will work out just fine (pause).

NOTE: Whether you'll be giving birth at home, in a birth center, or in a hospital, with a doctor or a midwife—and whether you call it "delivery" or "birthing"—it's all the same process, with the same magic. Don't get hung up on words. We've mixed up the language here and on the CD to reflect all your options. Feel free to translate!

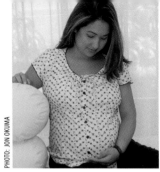

2. Now picture the faces of your doctor or midwife and nurses and others who will be attending you. They are greeting you with big smiles on friendly faces. You know they care about you and your baby and will be very supportive of your needs. You can hear them asking you questions to help make you comfortable. When you look at them you can feel their strength and their years of experience. A feeling of calm comes over you. You are protected and you know you are in good hands.

3. Now picture the faces of your family who have come to be with you on the big day. They are all there hugging you with their support. They are helping you feel assured of yourself and you know they will be there for you after baby is born. You can see the face of your partner or relative who will be staying with you, standing there right at your side. Maybe it's your midwife or a kind nurse holding your hand. You are not feeling afraid. Their hand gives you more strength and you can feel their love for you as they cheer you on. You are going to do just fine. You've come this far and your body knows exactly what to do.

4. Now the camera and the movie focuses on you. You can see yourself as you are in labor. You are very excited. You can see a slight smile on your face and inside you can feel a reserve of faith and confidence. You can handle this. You've got all these wonderful people helping you. You've carried and cared for your growing baby all these months and now you are ready. You can feel that inner strength and you know that your love for your baby will carry the day.

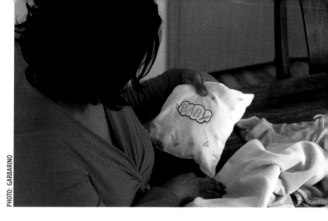

Week 35 Objective:

Use Quiet Time to prepare yourself for welcoming your baby.

My Pregnancy Journal

As you get closer to the big day write a letter to your baby, welcoming him into the world. Tell him what's going to happen and how it will feel to finally meet.

DEAR BABY _____ (name);
I wanted to let you know that I am getting our home ready for you by: _____

_____

You're due very soon now and I can hardly wait until:

_____

_____

I am going to be strong for you and help you have an easy birth because: _____

_____

My Pregnancy Journal, *continued*

When you are first born, here's what's going to happen:

_____

_____

_____

_____

_____

Then you're going to meet: _____

_____

_____

_____

_____

After that, I'm going to take care of you by: ____

Then we're going to take you home where you'll find: ____

_____

_____

_____

_____

_____

Week 36 Objective:

Use Quiet Time to create an affirmation for birth and welcoming baby.

YOUR BIRTH AFFIRMATION:

Create a statement of faith in yourself that you are becoming the best mother you can be. Find some powerful words that, when you say them, will remind you that you are fully capable of taking care of your new baby. Example: I'm ready to care for my baby.

I am:_____

_____

_____

(Say this out loud every day in front of the mirror when you get up and go to bed.)

Scenes of birth and bringing baby home: Your affirmation and last week's Quiet Time exercise have helped prepare you mentally for labor. Now you need to get ready to welcome baby into this world. This is the climactic end of a beautiful movie and the beginning of another featuring a new young star. Turn on the CD for selection 12 or have your partner read each scene below. Now get comfortable. Close your eyes, relax, breath deeply, and turn the projector on.

 Track 12

Scene 1: Giving Birth. Picture yourself getting ready to release your baby into the world. Your breathing is good; your contractions are strong. If it's a Cesarean, you are ready for that, too. Everyone is encouraging you. Baby is almost here. You feel a powerful urge. Then you feel a total release. There's a clamor. Oh my! The miracle of birth happens. You hear clapping and cheers. You've done it!

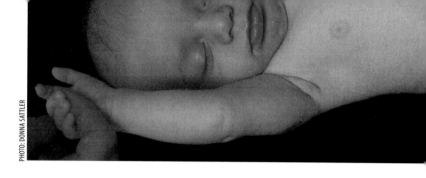

Scene 2: Meeting Baby. Now, for the first time, you feel your baby outside the womb. Your body has done its job. You feel his tiny weight on your chest as your arms wrap around him. You say hello and he seems to hear you and respond. Your partner sings his favorite song and baby looks to him. You both hold his tiny hands and you know this is your baby.

Scene 3: Feeding Baby. You're settling in after the excitement of delivery. You are feeling calm and happy and proud. You have just fed baby for the first time. You have taken in the smell of milk and the smell of your newborn. You have felt your body connect and move with your baby's soft steady sucking. Baby is sleeping now, safe in his mother's arms.

Scene 4: Bringing baby home. It felt like this day would never come, but you're standing at your doorstep bringing baby home. How beautiful this baby is, all bundled up snoozing in his little sack. You carry baby into the home you have prepared for him. You stand there just looking. Welcome home, baby.

You can continue to use the relaxation exercises and your affirmations and the pictures in your head to keep yourself strong and confident all the way up to your baby's birthday. Continue with a daily Quiet Time of any kind that you found particularly helpful. You'll want to keep taking that special time to just be with your baby for years to come.

 Track 13

Note: Ask your birth attendants to play "Symphony for Delivery" on track 13 of our CD (or other music that you've been playing for baby) in the birth room to calm you and baby. Ask one of your helpers to push "repeat" for about a half hour of music.

Week 37 and beyond Objective:
Relax and get ready for baby.

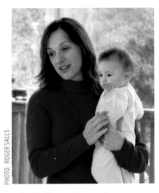

NOTE: The editors chose week 36 as the time to get ready for baby's birth because some babies can come at this age. But most moms will still have a month –or more—to go. Your relaxation habit will really help in the next few weeks.

Although you may not give birth for some time, we recommend repeating the exercises for week 35 and 36 and listening to tracks 11 and 12 on your CD to prepare mentally for the big day. In the meantime, here are some practical tips for preparing for other important things.

If you haven't already:

» **Go visit the place where you will give birth.** Seeing where you're going to have your baby will make you feel more comfortable when the time comes. What can you bring with you to make this place feel "just right" for you? Some flowers, or a photograph, or your own pillow?

» **Talk to your healthcare provider.** Share your plan for labor, birth, and afterwords with your doctor or midwife. Ask all your questions, and address any concerns you might have.

» **Make room for baby.** Get everything ready and safe for baby's homecoming including a car seat, clothes, and any needed supplies.

» **Prepare your family.** Get dad involved to help during labor and at home. Tell baby's brothers and sisters what's going to happen.

» **Arrange for some help at home.** You'll need time to focus on baby and rest. Some friendly advice will be nice, too!

» **Prepare for labor.** Prepare for labor. Find out about the signs of early labor, what to eat and drink and do during the early phases, and when to contact your midwife or doctor. Make a phone list of who to call. Pack your bag.

Congratulations and stay cool. You will soon have a beautiful baby – you're already a beautiful mother.

My Pregnancy Journal

Here's a chance to look back on your pregnancy and on the birth experience. Record thoughts and feelings now while they're fresh and full. You'll someday want to look back and share the first memories of being together.

THE PREGNANCY: The hardest part was: _____

_____

_____

What I enjoyed the most:_____

_____

_____

When I felt the closest to you: _____

_____

When I felt the closest to my partner: _____

_____

THE LABOR: The hardest part was: _____

_____

What gave me strength was: _____

_____

_____

The most exciting moment was when: _____

_____

_____

_____

_____

THE BIRTH: When I first saw you I thought: _____

_____

_____

_____

Our first moments together were like: _____

_____

_____

You seemed to react most to: _____

_____

_____

My feelings for you: _____

_____

_____

_____

My Pregnancy Journal _____

_____

_____

_____

_____

_____

_____

_____

_____

_____

_____

_____

_____

_____

_____

_____

_____

_____

_____

_____

_____

_____

_____

_____

My Pregnancy Journal _____

_____

_____

_____

_____

_____

_____

_____

_____

_____

_____

_____

_____

_____

_____

_____

_____

_____

_____

_____

_____

_____

_____

My Pregnancy Journal _____

_____

_____

_____

_____

_____

_____

_____

_____

_____

_____

_____

_____

_____

_____

_____

_____

_____

_____

_____

_____

My Pregnancy Journal _____

_____

_____

_____

_____

_____

_____

_____

_____

_____

_____

_____

_____

_____

_____

_____

_____

_____

_____

_____

_____

_____

My Pregnancy Journal _____

_____

_____

_____

_____

_____

_____

_____

_____

_____

_____

_____

_____

_____

_____

_____

_____

_____

_____

_____

_____

_____

My Pregnancy Journal

Recording Baby's movements (continued from page 50)

Do you ever feel a sharp kick or jump? _____

_____

When does that happen? _____

_____

Does baby's movement ever surprise you? _____

_____

Are there times when baby's movements hurt? _____

_____

Are there times when baby's movements feel good to you?_____

_____

Do baby's movements ever make you laugh? _____

_____

Do you ever sense when baby is changing positions? _____

_____

Can you ever tell where baby's head, feet, or bottom are? _____

_____

Does baby ever seem to move in a certain way depending on how
you feel?_____

Does your baby ever seem to
express feelings through movements? _____

_____

_____

_____

_____

_____

What do you think about that?

_____

_____

_____

_____

_____

**NOTE: AS PREGNANCY
PROGRESSES AND BABY'S
MOVEMENTS BECOME MORE
PRONOUNCED, YOU'LL
BECOME MORE SKILLED AT
SENSING THEM AND MAY
WANT TO COME BACK TO THESE
QUESTIONS.**

Partner's Pregnancy Journal

You're both in this together. The sooner you begin to think about your new role and talking things over with your partner, the better parent you'll become. Start by writing out your answers to these questions:

What did you think when you first found out your partner was pregnant? _____

_____

_____

_____

How do you think your life will change once baby is born? _____

_____

_____

Are there ways you can help support your partner? (Can you help her reduce her stress, listen to her better, do more around the house?) _____

_____

_____

_____

Are there any things you'd like to talk over with your partner? _____

_____

_____

What are some of the ways you can get involved now to prepare for parenthood? (such as learning about baby's development; attend prenatal visits and childbirth classes; get baby's room ready) _____

_____

_____

What did you think when you first felt the baby move in your partner's abdomen? _____

_____

_____

_____

Did you ever listen in to hear baby's heartbeat? What did you think? _____

_____

_____

Do you feel this baby will be like you in any way? How so? _____

_____

_____

How will you participate in baby's birth? _____

_____

_____

_____

More rhymes and songs

Humpty Dumpty

Humpty Dumpty sat on a wall.
Humpty Dumpty had a great fall.
All the king's horses and all the king's men
Couldn't put Humpty together again!

This Little Piggy Went to Market

This little piggy went to market,
This little piggy stayed home,
This little piggy had roast beef,
This little piggy had none,
And this little piggy cried,
 Wee, wee, wee, wee, wee,
All the way home.

The Teensy Weensy Spider

The Teensy Weensy Spider
Went up the water spout.
Down came the rain
And washed the spider out.
Out came the sun
And dried up all the rain.
And, the Teensy Weensy Spider
Went up the spout again.

You Are My Sunshine

You are my sunshine,
My only sunshine.
You make me happy
When skies are gray.
You'll never know dear,
How much I love you.
Please don't take
My sunshine away.

Jack and Jill

Jack and Jill went up the hill
To fetch a pail of water.
Jack fell down and broke his crown
And Jill came tumbling after.

Take Me Out to the Ballgame

Take me out to the ballgame.
Take me out to the crowd.
Buy me some peanuts and Cracker Jack,
I don't care if I ever come back.
So, it's root, root, root for the home team.
If they don't win it's a shame.
Oh, it's one, two, three strikes you're out
At the old ball game.

RESOURCES
for further learning
about the ideas introduced in this book:

» Peter Nathanielsz, M.D., PhD. The Prenatal Prescription. Harper Collins: New York. 2001.

» Thomas Verny, M.D. Nurturing the Unborn Child. Olmstead Press: Chicago. 2002.

» Thomas Verny, M.D. Pre-Parenting: Nurturing Your Child From Conception. Simon & Schuster: New York. 2002.

» Frederick Wirth, M.D. Prenatal Parenting. Harper Collins: New York. 2001.

» F. Rene van de Carr, M.D. and Marc Lehrer, While You're Expecting: Creating Your Own Prenatal Classroom. Humanics: Atlanta. 1996.

» Herbert Benson M.D. The Relaxation Response. Harper Collins: New York. 1976.

» Candace Pert, Ph.D. Molecules of Emotion: The Science Behind Mind-Body Medicine. Scribner: New York. 1999.

» Thomas Blum, Ph.D. (ed.) Prenatal Perception, Learning and Bonding. Leonardo: Berlin. 1993.

» T. Berry Brazelton, M.D. On Becoming a Family: The Growth of Attachment. Delacorte Press: New York. 1981.

» Association for Pre- & Perinatal Psychology and Health.
P.O. Box 1398, Forestville, CA 95436. www.birthpsychology.com

Some additional recources

» Healthy Families America
www.HealthyFamiliesAmerica.org

» American College of Nurse-Midwives
www.acnm.org

» La Leche League International
www.lalecheleague.org

» Lamaze International
www.lamaze.org

» www.askdoctorsears.com

» Doulas of North America
www.dona.org